The Keys To Healthy Living with Chronic Diseases for African Americans

A PRIMER FOR NUTRITION THERAPY IN THE PRIMARY CARE SETTING

Cheryl Campbell Atkinson

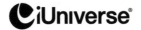

THE KEYS TO HEALTHY LIVING WITH CHRONIC DISEASES
A PRIMER FOR NUTRITION THERAPY

iUniverse books may be ordered through booksellers or by contacting:

iUniverse
1663 Liberty Drive
Bloomington, IN 47403
www.iuniverse.com
1-800-Authors (1-800-288-4677)

ISBN: 978-1-4917-4872-5 (sc)
ISBN: 978-1-4917-4873-2 (e)

Printed in the United States of America.

iUniverse rev. date: 11/18/2014

These basic guidelines have been prepared primarily
For use by
non-nutrition health care professionals.

INTENDED USER

A PROFESSIONAL RESOURCE MANUAL

The Keys to Healthy Living with Chronic Diseases for African Americans; A primer for nutrition therapy in the primary care setting is tailored to meet the varying educational backgrounds of most health care providers.

The nutrition therapy for the chronic diseases addressed in this book, namely Cancers, Diabetes, and Hypertension, sometimes referred to as the 'big three' are most appropriately designed and implemented by the skilled registered dietitian (RD). When an RD is not available, these responsibilities along with the subsequent monitoring of the patient will be the responsibility of a member of the health care team. This team member usually is a non-nutrition health professional.

A diagnosis of cancer, diabetes or hypertension can be devastating. This manual is designed to help the non-nutrition health professional obtain the basics necessary to provide initial counseling and/or monitoring of these patients, and in particular the African American patient with these nutrition related chronic illnesses.

The diet (also called the meal plan), which is included as part of the Nutrition therapy (NT) for the 'big three', parallels that of a moderate heart healthy plan, and must be strongly encouraged. The control of diabetes, hypertension and cancer works best when the meal plans are used in conjunction with the medical therapy, prescribed by the licensed physician.

This manual is a rich source of needed information for the non-nutrition health professional. This excellent counseling tool has been long needed in the public health primary care setting, and can be utilized by all health care professionals.

Lorna Shelton Beck MS, RD, CDE.

Table of Contents

Contributing Author

Vadel Shivers MS, RD, LDN, CSO
Oncology Dietitian
Mary Bird Perkins –Our Lady of the Lake Cancer Center
Baton Rouge, Louisiana

INTRODUCTION

THE AFRICAN AMERICAN PERSPECTIVE

The United States is a melting pot of many cultures from around the world. This cultural diversity impacts what and how we eat. Although African Americans now live in every State within the union, the lifestyle of parents and grandparents, who lived primarily in the southern United States, had the greatest influence on creating the social, religious and cultural traditions practiced by African Americans. These traditional practices, which have survived through today, have at their core, soul food cooking and gatherings with family and friends.

'Soul Food' is a term coined by African Americans to capture the uniqueness of the cooking style utilized for themselves, families and friends, all prepared with love, care and lots of soul. These foods differ from the more traditional southern foods in the use of plain ingredients, inexpensive cuts of meat, and seasonally grown or freshly caught foods. Many of the foods used are rich in healthful nutrients, however the cooking methods and the combination of typical food items used as flavoring/seasonings increases the sodium, fat and sugar content of traditional dishes to extremely high levels. African Americans have paid a high price for this lifestyle, with high incidences of cancer, diabetes and hypertension.

Most Americans eat too much salt in their daily diet, consuming up to twenty times the amount of salt needed by the body. Research suggests that diets high in salt (sodium) may cause an increase in blood pressure in many individuals. This is especially true in salt-sensitive individuals, such as African Americans. High blood cholesterol and high levels of saturated fat are also a risk factor for heart disease and certain cancers.. Fortunately, certain cancers, high blood pressure and diabetes can be controlled in part by making some simple changes in what you eat. Cutting back on salt and sodium can help lower blood pressure. Cutting back on saturated fat and cholesterol can help lower high blood cholesterol and impact certain cancers, and reducing carbohydrate intake can help control diabetes. It is also important to realize that eating fewer Kilocalories (kcal) will control overweight, obesity and several of the diet-related chronic diseases at the same time.

This manual provides the non-nutrition health-care professional with ideas to assist in planning the nutritional therapy for persons with dietary related chronic disease clients; cutting back on salt and carbohydrates, as well as providing soul food recipes that are lower in sodium, fat, sugar and cholesterol. It's all about 'heart-healthy living'.

SECTION ONE

USEFUL GUIDELINES FOR
THE
NUTRITIONAL
MANAGEMENT
OF
SELECT
CHRONIC DISEASES

DIABETES MELLITUS

PART - 1

DIABETES MELLITUS

FACTS AND FIGURES

Diabetes is the fourth leading cause of disease-related death for African Americans.

When compared to Caucasians, African Americans are 1.7 times more likely to have diabetes. Data from the American Diabetes Association indicates that approximately 2.3 million or 10.8% of all African Americans have diabetes, and about one-third of them are unaware that they have this deadly disease. The prevalence of this disease is striking in this ethnic group. It affects all age groups, but seems to have a high prevalence with persons from the age of fifty-five years and older. Twenty five percent, or one-out-of-four, in this age group have diabetes.

What is Diabetes?

Diabetes is a disease that affects the body's ability to produce or respond to insulin. Insulin is the hormone that allows blood glucose (also called blood sugar) to enter the cells of the body to be used for energy. Diabetes causes blood glucose to buildup in the body adversely affecting several organs of the body (kidneys, eyes, heart,) and normal body processes, and may lead to death. Almost all persons with diabetes can be considered to have insulin-dependent (IDDM) called Type 1, or non-insulin dependent (NIDDM) called Type 11. This disease is chronic, and has no cure.

- *Individuals with type 1 diabetes do not have the capabilities to produce insulin to help promote lower blood glucose levels. Those with type II diabetes can produce some insulin, but is it not properly used by the body or not enough is available to manage blood glucose in response to usual intake*

The complications that can be caused by diabetes are blindness, due to diabetic retinopathy; kidney disease due to diabetic nephropathy; heart disease and stroke; non-traumatic lower limb amputation; and impotence due to diabetic neuropathy or blood vessel blockage. Of these complications African Americans experience higher rates of blindness, kidney disease (failure), and amputation, than any other ethnic group.

CHAPTER 1

QUESTIONS ABOUT NUTRITION AND DIABETES

These are questions that the newly diagnosed diabetic may ask.

Q. *Can I eat foods with sugar in them?*

A. Yes! The truth is that sugar has gotten a bad reputation. Eating a slice of cake with sugar will raise blood sugar levels but so will eating corn on the cob, a tomato sandwich or red (kidney) beans. In the body they are all converted to glucose and used for energy. With sugary foods, the rule is moderation.

Q. *Does losing weight help my diabetes?*

A. Yes! First, it lowers insulin resistance. This allows natural insulin to do a better job lowering blood glucose levels. Second, it improves blood fat and blood pressure levels, reducing the risk of cardiovascular disease.

Q. *How much weight should I lose each week?*

A. Limiting your weight loss to one pound a week will keep you healthy and will keep the weight off. The general rule is: the faster you take it off, the faster it comes back on. A slow steady weight loss is the key to keeping weight off.

Q. *What foods can I eat a lot of?*

A. The key to healthy living is moderation. If you can control the portion of the food you eat, you will be able to eat a wider variety of foods, including your favorites, and still stick to your goals.

Q. *What can I do if I overeat over the holidays?*

A. Put on your walking shoes and head for the pavement. Spend the extra holiday hours making sure you take a thirty or forty five minute walk, once a day to help lower blood glucose levels.

Q. Can I use all the artificial sweetener I want?

A. Artificial (calorie-free) sweeteners like aspartame, saccharin, and acesulfame-K won't increase blood glucose level. These sweeteners are safe for everyone except pregnant or breastfeeding women, who should not use saccharin, and people with phenylketonuria, who should not use aspartame.

Q. Can I drink alcohol?

A. Yes, in moderation. Moderation is defined as two drinks a day for men and one drink a day for women. A drink is a 5-ounce glass of wine, a 12-ounce light beer, or 1-1/2 ounces of 80-proof distilled spirits. Make sure that the medications that you are currently taking **does not** recommend avoiding alcohol, and get your doctor's okay.

Q. Isn't glucose control easier if I eat the same things every day?

A. Probably, but it can become boring and it may not be nutritious. From a nutritional stand point, it is best to eat a variety of foods each day. By testing your blood glucose about an hour after meals, you will soon be able to predict what foods, and combinations of foods, raises your blood glucose levels.

Q. What vitamins will help my diabetes?

A. If you eat nutritiously, choosing a variety of fruits, vegetables, grains and meat each day, you wouldn't need to take vitamin supplements because of diabetes.

Q. Are there herbs that will help my diabetes?

A. Many herbs supposedly have glucose-lowering effects, but there are not enough data on any herb to recommend it for use in people with diabetes.

Q. Why do I need to see a dietitian?

A. Registered dietitians (RDs) have training and expertise in diabetes education and management, and are skilled in the coordination of diabetes medications and the diet. The RD will work with you to create a healthy eating plan that includes your favorite foods.

Source: Adapted from American Diabetes Association ; Nutrition FAQs

CHAPTER 2

NUTRITION ASSESSMENT

GENERAL GUIDELINES FOR
BASIC DIABETES NUTRITION THERAPY

Healthy eating is one of the basic and important diabetes care tools. Controlling diabetes through nutrition therapy can improve long–term health and the quality of life.

The goals of nutrition self-management for Diabetes Mellitus are:
1. to maintain as near-normal blood glucose levels, by balancing food, insulin and exercise;
2. to prevent hyperglycemia and hypoglycemia and,
3. to reduce the risk of atherosclerosis and microvascular complications.

Almost all persons with diabetes can be considered to have non-insulin dependent (NIDDM) or insulin-dependent (IDDM) The specific dietary recommendations and any additional considerations will vary based on type of diabetes and the medical management program, of which the nutrition therapy plays a major part.

The target blood glucose control ranges in Diabetes are:

* normal fasting plasma blood glucose: < 115 mg/dl
* normal post prandial plasma blood glucose   < 140 mg / dl
* normal glycosylate hemoglobin: HbAlc < 6 %

Non-insulin dependent diabetes mellitus and insulin dependent diabetes mellitus have distinctive features that are readily identifiable.

FEATURES OF IDDM AND NIDDM

	TYPE 1 (IDDM)	**TYPE 2 (NIDDM)**
Other names	Insulin dependent	Non-insulin dependent
	Juvenile-onset diabetes	Adult-onset diabetes
	Ketosis-prone diabetes	Ketosis-resistant diabetes
	Brittle diabetes	Stable diabetes
Age of onset	<20 (mean age, 12)	>40
Associated conditions	Viral infection, heredity	Obesity, heredity, aging
Insulin required?	Yes	Sometimes
Cell response to insulin	Normal	Resistant
Symptoms	Relatively severe	Relatively moderate
Prevalence in diabetic	5% to 10%	90% to 95%

Source: Nutrition for Health & Health Care

THE GLYCEMIC INDEX

The glycemic index is another tool that is useful in the teaching and counseling of the diabetic patients. The index measures how fast a food item is likely to raise blood sugar levels, and therefore can be helpful for managing sugars levels in the blood. The glycemic index is an indicator of the 'after-meal' response that the body has to a particular food compared to the reference standard, glucose; the fastest absorbed carbohydrate available. Glucose is given the value of one hundred (100) on the glycemic index, and other carbohydrates are given a number or an index relative to glucose.

Foods with a high glycemic index raise blood glucose faster and to a greater extent than foods with a low glycemic index. For example, if blood sugar levels tend to drop rapidly during exercise the consumption of a carbohydrate food that will raise blood sugar quickly (high glycemic index) is suggested. On the other hand, to help keep the blood sugar level as constant as possible during a few hours of mild activity, the consumption of a carbohydrate food that will raise blood sugar more slowly (lower glycemic index) is suggested. Carbohydrate foods with a lower glycemic index, also called slower carbs, are helpful for preventing overnight drops in the sugar level of the blood, and for long periods of exercise.

Since people are individuals and respond differently to metabolic changes, registered dietitians often encourage patients to monitor their blood sugar responses to carbohydrates foods, thereby creating their own individual glycemic index.

The Glycemic Index Range and a list of common carbohydrate foods with the corresponding index are provided below:

Glycemic Index Range

Low Glycemic Index	=	55 or less
Medium Glycemic Index	=	56 – 69
High Glycemic Index	=	70 or more

**REMEMBER:

The glycemic index is an additional tool what works together with the patient's current meal planning system to successfully control daily blood glucose (sugar) levels.

Glycemic Index Guide : Examples of Foods by Categories

FOOD CATEGORIES	INDEX	FOOD CATEGORIES	INDEX
CEREALS		**FRUIT**	
All Bran	51	Apple	38
Cheerios	74	Banana	56
Cornflakes	83	Grapefruit	25
Life	66	Mango	55
Oatmeal, old fashion	48	Peach	42
Raisin Bran	73	Watermelon	72
SNACKS		**CRACKERS**	
Chocolate Bar	49	Graham crackers	74
Croissant	67	Rice cakes	80
Doughnut	76	Pretzels	83
Pizza Hut, supreme	33	Soda crackers, saltines	72
Pound Cake	54	Wheat thins	67
Oatmeal Cookies	55	Rye	68
GRAINS		**SUGARS/CANDIES**	
Barley	25	Fructose	22
Basmati white Rice	58	Honey	62
Brown Rice	55	Table sugar (sucrose)	64
Instant White Rice	87	Glucose Tablets	102
Couscous	65	Jelly Beans	80
Cornmeal	68	M&M chocolate candies	33

PASTA		VEGETABLES	
Fettuccini	32	Carrot	49
Macaroni	45	Green Pea	47
Macaroni and Cheese	64	Lima Beans	32
Dinner	33	Corn	56
Spaghetti	50	Parsnips	97
Cheese Tortellini	35	Tomato	38
Vermicelli			

FOOD CATEGORIES	**INDEX**	**FOOD CATEGORIES**	**INDEX**
BEANS/ROOT CROPS		**BREADS**	
Baked beans	48	Bagel, plain	72
Kidney beans	52	Croissant	67
Black beans	30	Blueberry muffin	59
Chickpeas (garbanzo	33	White, sliced	70
beans)	54	Whole wheat	68
Sweet potatoes	70	Pumpernickel, whole	49
White potatoes (Irish)		grain	

DRINKS		**MILK PRODUCTS**	
Apple juice	40	Whole milk	30
Colas (sodas)	65	Chocolate milk	35
Gatorade	78	Skim milk	32
Grapefruit juice	48	Soy milk	31
Orange juice	46	Ice cream	60
Pineapple juice	46	Yogurt, fruit	36

Steps To Incorporating a Low Glycemic Index Diet

The use of the glycemic index meal planning tool can be introduced to the patient through a series of recommendations. Recommend that patients;

- Use breakfast cereals based on oats, barley and bran
- Use 'grainy' bread made with whole seeds
- Reduce the amount of white potatoes
- Reduce the amount of white rice
- Enjoy all types of fruit and vegetables (except potatoes)
- Eat plenty of salad vegetables with vinaigrette dressing

Source: modified from Home of the Glycemic Index. ***www.glycemicindex.com****; and Food and Diet in Diabetes.* ***www.Diabetesnet.com***

CHAPTER 3

DIETARY RECOMMENDATIONS

The nutrition therapy that is used as part of the management of diabetes mellitus is controlled in kilocalories (kcalories, but more often written as calories), proteins, fat and carbohydrate. The specific dietary recommendations or meal plan will vary with the type of diabetes mellitus and with the total medical management program as prescribed by the doctor or primary health care provider, and the registered dietitian.

KILOCALORIES
Following the American Diabetes Association guidelines:

12 – 20 %	of kcalories should come from	- protein
20 – 30 %	of kcalories	- fat
55 - 60 %		- carbohydrate

to;
* achieve and maintain healthy body weight
* achieve normal growth and development
* to meet increased demands during pregnancy and lactation

CARBOHYDRATES
Following the American Diabetes Association guidelines:

55 – 60 %   of kcalories should come from   - carbohydrates

Although various starches have different glycemic responses, from a clinical perspective, the total amount of carbohydrate consumed is more important that the source of type of carbohydrate.
-   individualized based on the persons eating habits
-   distribution of carbohydrates in the meal pattern will vary with insulin regimens and treatment goals.

PROTEIN

Following the American Diabetes Association guidelines:

10 – 20 %   of kcalories should come from   - protein

The RDA protein intake (0.8 g/kg body weight) for persons with diabetes is similar to non- diabetic persons.

FAT

Following the American Diabetes association guidelines:

20 – 30%   of kilocalories   should come from   - fat

note;

< 10%   of kilocalories   should come from   - saturated fat
60 – 70%   of kilocalories   should come from   - mono unsaturated fats

If obesity and weight loss are the primary concern, dietary fat intake must be reduced.

ALCOHOL

The consumption of Alcoholic beverages is not recommended for persons with diabetes. Like sugar, alcohol provided empty kcalories, and a high intake of alcoholic beverages may cause several health problems. Alcohol may have a hypoglycemic effect on persons with diabetes.

Simple alternatives may be club soda with lemon or lime, diet sodas or sparkling (non-kcaloric) water.

CHAPTER 4

GENERAL NURITION PROTOCOLS

A) IDDM OR TYPE-1 DIABETES

GOAL:
To maintain day-to-day consistency in the timing and amount of food intake in persons receiving conventional Insulin therapy.

GUIDELINES:
- **Consume adequate kilocalories to maintain healthy weight.**
  (Kilocalorie [Kcalorie] intake for the meal plan should be determined by the primary healthcare provider. example: MD, RN or RD. Whenever possible, the dietitian RD, should provide diet instructions.)

- Keep the timing of meals consistent from day to day, and synchronized with the time-actions of insulin.
  It is not necessary to provide meals and snacks into any artificial or unnatural division. Stay as close as possible to the usually eating pattern of the individual.

- Depending upon the insulin regimen, plan a bedtime snack to prevent nocturnal hypoglycemia.

EXAMPLE OF DAILY MEAL PLAN:

(all meal plans should be individualized based on the assessment and evaluation of the patient's condition)

If an individual is receiving conventional Insulin therapy;

> 3 meals per day   (spaced 4-5 hours apart)
> bedtime snack

therefore;

> Inject AM insulin   ½ hour before breakfast
> Other insulin   ½ hour before meal

Or at designated evening time

Usually only 15 gm of carbohydrate (1 starch exchange), and 1 oz of protein (1 exchange) are needed for a bedtime snack.

Example of 15 gm carbohydrate: -
- 4 ozs. apple / orange juice
- 10 ozs. milk
- 3 graham crackers
- 6 saltine crackers
- 3 glucose tablets
- 4 life savers (hard candy)

Example of 1 ounce protein: -
- 8 ozs. milk
- 1 carton yogurt
- (w/ NutraSweet)
- 1 oz. Cheese
- 1 egg
- 2 Tablespoons Peanut butter

* Limit simple carbohydrate to 10% -15% of total kcalories:

Simple Carbohydrates: defined as mono and disaccharides which are lactose, sucrose and fructose.

        Example: Table sugar
                    Corn syrup
                    Honey
                    Molasses

- Make modifications in the dietary management plan for hypertension, hyperlipidemia and / or renal insufficiency.

  Eat salt and sodium in moderation. Do not advise the use of any commercially prepared or seasoned meats, entrees, vegetables, potatoes, macaroni or rice dishes.

Limit fried foods to only one time every other week (biweekly). Fats, such as margarine mayonnaise, salad dressings should be used sparingly -1 teaspoon/ per serving.

- If obesity or overweight is present, follow a low kcalorie diet to reduce and maintain a desirable weight.

  Regular exercise is of primary importance in achieving desirable weight.

NOTE: Advise all patients to consult a doctor before starting any exercise regime.

- Test blood glucose 2- 4 times daily.

TREATMENT FOR HYPOGLYCEMIA

If Hypoglycemia occurs the <u>15:15 Rule</u> should be applied

RULE:

TAKE **15** GRAMS OF FAST ACTING SUGAR
WAIT **15** MINUTES THEN CHECK BLOOD LEVELS
IF GREATER THAN 70 MG %---EAT SNACK OR MEAL
BUT;
IF LESS THAN 70 MG % ----REPEAT THE 15:15 RULE

********* 15 Grams of carbohydrate should increase blood
sugar by 30 mg % in 15 minutes ********

B) NIDDM OR TYPE-11 DIABETES

<u>GOAL:</u>
To follow an appropriate dietary regime, that will best achieve a satisfactory
(acceptable) blood glucose levels.

GUIDELINES:

*   **Eat well- balanced meals, including: Protein, Starch,
    Vegetables and Fruit.**

Example:	3ozs. meat	= the size of a deck of cards
	starches	= rice, potatoes, breads, and starchy vegetables <u>ex.</u> beans, peas, and corn,
	vegetables	= broccoli, green beans, cabbage. Carrots
	fruits	= fresh, canned fruit or juice.

- Keep the timing of the meals and the composition of the diet consistent from day to day.
  Spread the nutrients throughout the day, instead of only in three meals.

When eating fruit or drinking fruit juice, always have it with a meal or snack, never on an empty stomach. REMEMBER ; never drink more than 4 ozs. (1/2 cup) of juice at one time.

- A kilocalorie-restricted diet (sometimes referred to as a low calorie diet) must be followed if obesity is present.

<u>Rule of Thumb:</u>

A moderate kcalorie- restricted diet is one that has 250-500 kcalories less daily, than the usual daily intake.

- Limit simple carbohydrate to 10% - 15% of the total kcalories
  Simple Carbohydrates: defined as mono., and disaccharides which are lactose, sucrose and fructose.
  Example: table sugar
  Corn syrup
  Honey
  Molasses
  Sorghum

- The carbohydrate content (bread exchange) should be evenly divided from meal to meal
  Avoid concentrated sweets: candy, colas, doughnuts, ketchup etc.
  Drink diet beverages only: Use an artificial sweetener in coffee, tea or lemonade etc.

- **Regular exercise is of primary importance in achieving desirable weight.**
  Even a moderate weight loss (10-20 pounds) has been shown to improve diabetes control.

NOTE: Consult a doctor before starting any exercise regime.

- Plan a bedtime snack to prevent nocturnal hypoglycemia when either a short or long acting hypoglycemia agent is used. (chlorpropamide, glyburide, acetohexamide, tolbutamide, tolazamide, glipzide etc.)

Usually only 15 gm of carbohydrate (1starch exchange), and 1 oz of protein (1 exchange) are needed for a bedtime snack.

Example of 15 gm carbohydrate:-   4 ozs. apple/ orange juice
                                    10 ozs. milk
                                    3 grahams crackers
                                    5 saltine crackers
                                    4 glucose tablets
                                    5 life savers (hard candy)

Example of 1 ounce protein:-   8 ozs. milk
                                    1 carton yogurt (w/NutraSweet)
                                    1 oz. Cheese
                                    1 egg
                                    2 tablespoons Peanut butter

- Test blood glucose 2-4 times daily.

TREATMENT FOR HYPOGLYCEMIA

If Hypoglycemia occurs the <u>15:15 Rule</u> should be applied

RULE:

TAKE 15 GRAMS OF FAST ACTING SUGAR

WAIT 15 MINUTES THEN CHECK BLOOD LEVELS

IF GREATER THAN CHECK 70 MG %---- EAT SNACK OR MEAL

BUT;

IF LESS THAN 70 MG % --- REPEAT THE 15: 15 RULE

******** 15 Grams of carbohydrate should increase blood
sugar by 30 mg % in 15 minutes. ***********

Modifications in the "Soul Food Diet" in NIDDM

The traditional diet of most African Americans follow closely the 'traditional soul food diet' which utilized fried foods, saturated fat and high-fat products, exacerbating obesity and the risk factors for diabetes.

The information provided below is useful when counseling the African American patient.

General recommendations:

The amount and type of fat must be modified to encourage healthy caloric intake and to prevent the risk of obesity, and associated health factors. Correct portion sizes must be strictly maintained, and the consumption of a meatless main dish at least twice per week, should be encouraged, to promote health weight. Emphasize the benefits of whole grain products, fresh fruits and vegetables and the use of acceptable alternative sweeteners.

<u>Foods to be avoided:</u>	<u>Foods that can be used:</u>
High-fat meats;	
Chicken wings	Vegetable / Olive oil
Bologna	skin-free turkey necks
Sausages	liquid smoke (for flavor)
Fried Meats	margarine
Lard	egg whites
Ham hocks	fat-free broth
Bacon grease	
Simple Carbohydrates;	
White bread	whole wheat, whole grain bread
Cakes	whole wheat pasta
Pies	beans, peas

White (flour) pasta	sugar-free dessert products:
Soft drinks	Soft drinks
Ice Cream	Ice cream
	Yogurt
	Pudding
	Cake

Source: Modified from 'Ethnic and regional Food practices: Soul and Traditional Southern Food Practices, Customs, and Holiday'

CHAPTER 5

DIETARY MANAGEMENT

CARBOHYDRATE COUNTING

During the past decade a paradigm shift has occur in Diabetes Management. Priority is being given to ***the total amount of carbohydrate*** consumed at each meal and at snack time, rather than the ***source*** of the carbohydrate. When an individual with diabetes has the ability to control their daily carbohydrate intake, they are better able to manage their blood glucose levels. Carbohydrates affect the glucose levels in blood more than protein or fat.

To be competent with carbohydrate counting, patients must first understand the exchange list system and establish healthy eating habits, use correct portion sizes, and learn to eat consistent amount of carbohydrate at regular times. Where possible the services of a dietitian or nutritionist should be used because they are best trained health care professional to offer assistance with calculating the carbohydrates and calories that are appropriate for each diabetic patient.

RULE of THUMB:
  About half (50%) of the kcalories intake should be carbohydrates (carbs).
  There are about 4 calories in every gram of carbohydrates.

REMEMBER

Example:

    With a meal plan of 1200 calories a day
    About 600 calories should be from carbohydrates
    600 divided by 4   = 150 carb grams daily
    Daily goal   = 150 grams

Formula:

$$\frac{(calories/2)}{4} = \text{carb grams per day}$$

Once the goal for carbohydrate is established it becomes essential that the diabetic individual learns to determine the amount of carbohydrates in various portion sizing of food. Routine use of the *Food Facts Label*, and using the *Exchange List for Meal Planning* will help to determine and monitor total carbohydrate intake.

Remember:

When using the exchange system, one starch exchange equals about 15 grams of carbohydrate. One milk exchange is about 12 grams, and a vegetable exchange is about 15 grams.

To use this system effectively the common measuring units used by the patient must be reviewed and completely understood.

COMMON MEASUREMENTS:

3 teaspoons (tsp.)	=	1 tablespoon (Tbsp.)
4 tablespoons (Tbsps.)	=	¼ cup
5 1/3 tablespoons (Tbsps.)	=	1/3 cup
4 ounces (ozs.)	=	½ cup
8 ounces (ozs.)	=	1 cup
1 cup	=	½ pint

The advantages of this technique include more precise matching of food and insulin, greater flexibility with food choices, and an improved potential for success with food intake and improved blood glucose control.

CHAPTER 6

THE FOOD EXCHANGE LIST

WHAT ARE THE EXCHANGE LISTS?

They are lists of foods that are grouped together because they have about the same amount of carbohydrate, protein fat and kcalories. In the amounts given, any food on a list can be exchanged, traded or swapped for any other food on the same list. Several foods, such as beans and peas are on two lists.

The complete listing of the United States Exchange Lists, can be obtained for patient use, from the web site of the American Dietetic Association and the American Diabetic Association.

Example of the Exchange list

VEGETABLES:
Contain 25 calories and 5 grams of carbohydrates. One serving equals:

½ cup	Cooked vegetables (carrots, broccoli, zucchini, cabbage)
1 cup	Raw vegetables or salad greens
½ cup	Vegetable Juice

FAT-FREE and LOWFAT MILK:
Contain 90 calories. One serving equals:

1 cup	Milk, fat-free or 1% fat
¾ cup	Yogurt, plain non-fat or low fat
1 cup	Yogurt, artificially sweetener

VERY LEAN PROTEIN:

Contain 35 calories and 1 gram fat per serving. One serving equals:

1 ounce	Turkey or Chicken breast
1 ounce	Fisk fillet
1 ounce	Canned tuna in water
1 ounce	Shellfish (clams, lobster, scallop, shrimp)
¾ cup	Cottage cheese, non-fat or low fat
2 each	Egg whites
¼ cup	Egg substitute
1 ounce	Fat-free cheese
½ cup	Beans – cooked (black beans, kidney, chick peas or lentils): count as 1 starch/bread and 1 very lean protein.

LEAN PROTEIN:

Contains 55 calories and 2-3 grams of fat per serving. One serving equals:

1 ounce	Chicken - dark meat
1 ounce	Turkey – dark meat
1 ounce	Salmon, Swordfish, Herring
1 ounce	Lean beef
1 ounce	Veal, Roast or Lean chop*
1 ounce	Lamb, Roast or Lean chop*
1 ounce	Pork, tenderloin or fresh ham*
¼ cup	4.5% cottage cheese
2 medium	Sardines

MEDIUM FAT PROTEINS:

Contains 75 calories and 5 grams of fat per serving. One serving equals:

1 ounce	Beef (any prime cut), corned beef, ground beef**
1 ounce	Pork chop
1 each	Whole egg (medium)**
1 ounce	Mozzarella cheese
¼ cup	Ricotta cheese
4 ounces	Tofu

FRUITS:

Contain 15 grams of carbohydrates and 60 calories. One serving equals:

1 small	Apple, banana, orange, nectarine
1 medium	Fresh peach
1	Kiwi
½	Grapefruit
½	Mango
1 cup	Fresh berries (strawberries, raspberries or blueberries)
1 cup	Fresh melon cubes
1/8th	Honeydew melon
4 ounces	Unsweetened Juice
4 teaspoons	Jelly or Jam

STARCHES:

Contains 75 calories and 5 grams fat. One serving equals:

1 slice	Bread (white, pumpernickel, whole wheat, rye)
2 slice	Reduced calorie or 'lite' Bread
¼ (1 ounce)	Bagel
½	English muffin
½	Hamburger bun
¾ cup	Cold cereal
1/3 cup	Rice, brown or white
1/3 cup	Barley or Couscous
1/3 cup	Legumes
½ cup	Pasta

MEAL PLANNING

The meal plan is a guide, which shows the number of food choices or exchanges available at each meal and at snack time.

NOTE:

IT IS RECOMMENDED THAT A DIETITIAN OR NUTRITIONIST (RDN) DESIGN THE MEAL PLAN BASED ON INDIVIDUAL NEEDS.

MEAL PLANS:
The table below shows sample meal plans for different kilocalorie levels. The kilocalorie levels are usually prescribed by the attending doctor.

	1,200	1,500	1,800	2,000	2,500	Other: ____
Carbohydrates	(11)	(13)	(16)	(17)	(22)	
Starch	5	7	8	9	11	
Fruit	3	3	4	4	6	
Milk	2	2	3	3	3	
Vegetables	2	2	3	4	5	
Other						
Meat & Meat Substitutes	4	4	6	6	8	
Fat	3	4	4	5	6	

Explanation:

The numbers that are displayed throughout the table reflect the number of exchanges (measured portions) from each food group available daily on a specific meal plan.

A 1,200 kcalorie meal plan has 11 exchanges of carbohydrates. This includes 5 exchanges from starch, 3 from fruit, 2 from milk and 2 from starchy vegetables. Four (4) exchanges will come from meat and 3 exchanges will come from fat.

Example of Sample Menu for a day
This is a 1,200 kcalorie meal plans with 10-11 carbohydrate exchanges.

Breakfast: 1 scrambled egg

1 buttermilk biscuit (1 carbohydrate)

1 tsp. margarine

½ grapefruit section (1 carbohydrate)

8 fl. oz. skim milk (1 carbohydrate)

Lunch: 1 cup macaroni & cheese (2)

½ cup carrot sticks

½ cup celery sticks

2 Tbsp. dip

1 cup melon (1)

diet soda

Dinner: ½ cup red beans and rice (1)

2 ozs cornbread (1)

½ cup cooked greens

1 tsp. olive oil

½ cup canned peaches (1)

8 fl. ozs skim milk (1)

Source: adapted from 'Eating Right When You Have Diabetes'.

CHAPTER 7

DIET –DRUG INTERACTIONS

Medications (also called Drugs) can be used to help control blood pressure. These oral antidiabetic agents must not be used to replace diet and physical activity in the management of diabetes. Patients must be advises to continue their medical nutritional therapy. People with type 1 diabetes need to utilize insulin to control blood glucose while people with type 2 diabetes need to utilize a combination of diet and physical activity to maintain blood pressure within normal limits. Oral antidiabetic medications are taken by mouth to assist with the lowering of blood glucose levels in people with type 2 diabetes.

The effects of drugs on the diet of the diabetic patient are often subtle, slow to appear and at times, hard to recognize. Foods can make a medication more or less powerful, and drugs can interfere with the body's ability to absorb nutrients from food. Drugs may also affect nutrition by causing loss of appetite, dry mouth, nausea, diarrhea or constipation.

The list below contains information about common interactions that may occur between food and drugs that may be taken for diabetes. It does not attempt to discuss all possible food-drug interactions, nor does it list possible drug-drug interactions.

<u>Diet-Drug Interactions</u>

Insulin:
The timing of *insulin* administration varies, depending on the
Action of the insulin prescribed. Insulin may cause hypoglycemia.

Alpha-Glucosidase Inhibitors (Acarbose and Meglitol):
Alpha-Glucosidase Inhibitors are taken at the start of each meal.
Clients using these agents must use glucose to treat hypoglycemia.
Nutrition-related side effects include abdominal pain, gas and diarrhea.

Lispro (Insulin Analog):

Lispro is taken 5 to 10 minutes before meals. Lispro lowers the risk of hypoglycemia compared to insulin.

Metformin:

Metformin is taken once or twice a day before meals (breakfast or breakfast and dinner). GI side effects are uncommon, but metformin may cause diarrhea or leave a metallic taste in the mouth.

Nateglinide:

Nateglinide is taken immediately before eating. Nateglinide can cause hypoglycemia and sometimes diarrhea.

Repaglinide:

Repaglinide is taken before meals. Repaglinide can cause hypoglycemia and diarrhea.

Sulfonylureas (Chlorpropamide, Glipzide, Glyburide, Glimepiride):

Sulfonylureas are generally taken one or two times a day, before Meals. Disulfiram-like reactions can occur when large amounts of alcohol are taken (especially with chlorpropamide). These medications can also cause hypoglycemia.

Thioglitazones (Rosiglitazone, Piolitazone):

Thioglitazones are taken once or twice a day before meals. Nutrition Related side effects are uncommon. One medication of this type, Troglitazone, was recently taken off the market due to concerns that its use might be a cause of liver failure.

This is only a partial list of the most common medications available. It is strongly recommended that you consult with a Pharmacist or the MD regarding usage and side- effects of any medication.

Source: Adapted from 'Understanding Normal and Clinical Nutrition" sixth Edition.

CHAPTER 8

USEFUL TERMS

Diabetes-related terms that are importance in understanding and counseling African American patients in understanding their disease.

50/50 Insulin:
Premixed insulin that is fifty percent (50%) intermediate acting (NPH) insulin and fifty percent (50%) short-acting or regular insulin.

70/30 Insulin:
Premixed insulin that is seventy percent (70%) intermediate acting [NPH] insulin and thirty percent (30%) short-acting or regular insulin.

A1C:
Also called glycosylated hemoglobin or hemoglobin A1C, is a test that measures a person's average blood glucose level over the past 2 to 3 months. The test shows the amount of glucose that sticks to the red blood cell, which is proportional to the amount of glucose in the blood.

ACE Inhibitor:
An oral medicine that lowers blood pressure; Ace stands for 'angiotensin converting enzyme'. For people with diabetes, especially those who have protein (albumin) in the urine, it also helps slow down kidney damage.

Aspartame:
A dietary sweetener with almost no calories and no nutritional value. (Brand names; Equal, NutraSweet)

Blood Glucose:
The main sugar found in the blood and the body's main source of energy. Also called Blood sugar.

Blood Glucose level:
The amount of glucose in a given amount of blood. It is noted in milligrams in a deciliter, or mg/dl.

Blood Urea Nitrogen (BUN):
A waste product in the blood from the breakdown of protein. The kidneys filter blood to remove urea. As kidney function decreases, the BUN levels increase.

Body Mass Index (BMI):
A measure used to evaluate body weigh relative to a person's height. BMI is used to find out if a person is underweight, normal weight, overweight or obese.

Borderline Diabetes:
A former term for Type 2 diabetes or impaired glucose tolerance.

Brittle Diabetes:
A term used when a person's blood glucose level moves often from low to high and from high to low.

Carbohydrate Counting:
A method of meal planning for people with diabetes based on counting the number of grams of carbohydrate in food.

Creatinine: Le Lepp
A waste product from protein in the diet and from the muscles of the body. Creatinine is removed from the body by the kidney; as kidney disease progresses, the level of Creatinine in the blood increases.

Diabetic Ketoacidosis (DKA):
An emergency condition in which extremely high blood glucose levels, along with a severe lack of insulin, result in the breakdown of body fat for energy and an accumulation of ketones in the blood and urine. Signs of DKA are nausea and vomiting, stomach pain, fruity breath odor and rapid breathing. Untreated DKA can lead to coma and death.

Diabetic Nephropathy:
Disease of the kidney: Hyperglycemia and hypertension can damage the kidneys' glomeruli. When the kidneys are damaged, protein leaks out of the kidneys into the urine. Damaged kidneys can no longer remove waste and extra fluids from the bloodstream.

Diabetic Neuropathy:
Disease of the nervous system. The three major forms in people with diabetes are peripheral neuropathy, autonomic neuropathy, and mononeuropathy. The most common form is peripheral neuropathy, which affects mainly the legs and feet.

Diabetic Retinopathy:
Diabetic eye disease; damage to the small blood vessels in the retina. Loss of vision may result.

Exchange List:
One of several tools for diabetes meal planning. Foods are placed into three groups based on their nutritional content. Lists provide the serving sizes for carbohydrates meat and meat alternatives and fats. These lists allow for substitution for different groups to keep the nutritional content fixed.

Fasting Blood Glucose Test:
A check of a person's blood glucose level after the person has not eaten for 8 to 12 hours (usually overnight). This test is used to diagnose pre-diabetes and diabetes. It is also used to monitor people with diabetes.

Gestational Diabetes Mellitus (GDM):
A type a diabetes mellitus that develops only during pregnancy and usually disappears upon delivery, but increases the risk that the mother will develop diabetes later. GDM is managed with meal planning, activity and, in some cases, insulin.

Glaucoma:
An increase in fluid pressure inside the eye that may lead to loss of vision.

Glycemic Index:
A ranking of carbohydrate-containing foods, based on the food's effect on blood glucose compared with a standard reference food.

Hyperglycemia:
Excessive blood glucose: Fasting hyperglycemia is blood glucose above a desirable level after a person has fasted for at least 8 hours. Postprandial hyperglycemia is blood glucose above a desirable level 1 to 2 hours after a person has eaten.

Hypoglycemia:
A condition that occurs when one's blood glucose is lower than normal, usually less than70mg/dl. Signs include hunger, nervousness, shakiness, perspiration, dizziness or light-headedness, sleepiness and confusion. If left untreated, hypoglycemia may lead to unconsciousness.

Juvenile Diabetes:
Former term for Insulin-dependent diabetes (IDDM), or Type 1 diabetes.

Ketone:
A chemical produced when there is a shortage of insulin the blood and the body breaks down body fat for energy. High levels of ketones can lead to diabetic Ketoacidosis and coma. Sometimes referred to as ketone bodies.

Urine testing:
Also called 'urinalysis' – A test of a urine sample to diagnose diseases of the urinary system and other body systems. Urine may also be checked for signs of bleeding. Some tests use a single urine sample. For others, 24-hour collection may be needed.

Xylitol:
A carbohydrate-based sweetener found in plants and used as a substitute for sugar; provides calories. Found in some mints and chewing gum.

Source: Adopted from Diabetes Information Library: Diabetes-Related Definitions

<u>REFERENCES</u>

Diabetes Among African Americans. American Diabetes Association
<u>www.diabetes.org/ada/facts</u> . Retrieved (2010)

Diabetic Recipes. <u>www.diabetessymptom.net</u> Retrieved (2011)

Diabetes Care. 2012 Feb;35(2):305-12. doi: 10.2337/dc11-1405. Epub
2011 Dec 21.
<u>Cultural issues in **diabetes**. Dietary counseling for black patients.</u>
Vorderstrasse AA.

Cataldo, C. B., DeBruyne, L. K., Whitney, E, N. *Nutrition and Diet
Therapy: Principles and Practice.* Wadworth/Thomson Learning, 2003

Counting Calories and Carbos. Novo Nordisk Pharmaceuticals Inc., 1998

Ethnic and Regional Food Practices, A Series. *Soul and Traditional
Southern Food Practices, Customs, and Holidays.* The American Dietetic
Association, & The Diabetes Association, Inc. (1995)

Ewing, J., *Cultural Diversity: Eating in American, African American*
HYG-5250-95
<u>www.ohioline.osu.edu</u> Retrieved (2004)

Food & Diet in Diabetes. *Glycemic Index. How quickly do foods raise your
blood sugar?* <u>www.diabetesnet.com</u> Retrieved (2004)

Food and Drug Interactions. Munson Army Health Center. 2001
<u>www.munson.amedd.army.mil</u>. Retrieved (2004)

Frequently asked Questions: Nutrition and Diabetes. American Diabetes
Association 2000. <u>www.diabetes.org/nutirtion/faqs.asp</u>. Retrieved (2004)

Heart Smart Cookbook. Henry Ford Heart & Vascular Institute and The
Detroit Free Press. (1995)

Joslin Diabetes Center. *What is the Glycemic Index and Is It a Helpful Tool?* www.joslin.harvard.edu Retrieved (2011)

Lynch EB, Liebman R, Ventrelle J, Avery EF, Richardson D. A self-management intervention for African Americans with comorbid diabetes and hypertension: a pilot randomized controlled trial. Prev Chronic Dis. 2014;11:E90

National Heart, Lung, and Blood Institute. *Food Exchange List.* www.nhlbi.nih.gov Retrieved (2011)

Powers, M., *Guide To Eating Right When You Have Diabetes; The Comprehensive approach to Managing your Diabetes by eating well.* American Dietetic Association 2003.

Single-Topic Diabetes Resources. The American Dietetic Association, & The Diabetes Association, Inc. (1995)

Whitney, E. N., Cataldo, C.B., Rolfes, S.R. *Understanding Normal and Clinical Nutrition.* Seven Edition. Wadworth/Thomson Learning Inc. 2009.

Effects of food-related interventions for **African** American women with type 2 **diabetes.**
Sumlin LL, Garcia AA. **Diabetes** Educ. 2012 Mar-Apr;38(2):236-49. doi: 10.1177/0145721711422412. Review.

A systematic literature review of **diabetes** self-management **education** features to improve **diabetes education** in women of Black **African/** Caribbean and Hispanic/Latin American ethnicity. Gucciardi E, Chan VW, Manuel L, Sidani S.

Patient Educ Couns. 2013 Aug;92(2):235-45. doi: 10.1016/j. pec.2013.03.007. Epub 2013 Apr 6. Review.

Racial/ethnic- and **education**-related disparities in the control of risk factors for cardiovascular disease among individuals with **diabetes**. Chatterji P, Joo H, Lahiri K. Adv NPs PAs. 2010 Nov;1(3):26-9; quiz 30. No abstract available

CANCERS

PART 2
CANCERS
Prepared by Vadel Shivers MS, RD and Cheryl Atkinson PhD, RD

CANCER: WHAT IS IT?

Cancer is an uncontrollable growth of cells that destroys the function of normal cells (3). Normal cells can no longer function correctly causing changes in the way the body uses carbohydrates, fats, and proteins. If cancer is allowed to progress, it can quickly spread to major organs, bone, or vital tissues, impair normal function, and lead to death if not treated.

Focus on African Americans
While cancer affects individuals without regard to race, it appears to affect African-Americans severely, causing the highest rate of death and shortest survival of any racial and ethnic group. Research studies suggest that African-Americans have a greater incidence of developing major cancers and are twice as likely to die of a major cancer compared to whites (1). Factors such as limited knowledge and misinformation about cancer, mistrust of the medical community, concerns about privacy, lack of insurance, religious beliefs, and fear contribute to the increasing presence of cancer within the African American population (1b).

In an effort to reduce the incidence of cancer within the African-American community, education, early screening, and effective nutrition counseling needs to be easily accessible. Successful intervention is usually achieved when culturally sensitive information, and treatment are provided. Nutrition screening and counseling by a dietitian (RD) should be required protocol in the treatment of all chronic health conditions, especially cancer.

The Most Frequently occurring Cancer in African-Americans
Many factors play a major role in the increased development of cancer. Factors including poor eating or dietary habits, chewing tobacco use, cigarette smoking, and age may significantly contributed to the development of this disease.

Listed below are some of the risk factors associated with specific cancer types:

Breast Cancer - Linked to;
- Over consumption of alcoholic drinks
- Abdominal body fatness, overweight and obesity
- Inadequate physical activity
- Not bearing children or late pregnancy (over age 30)
- Late natural menopause
- Use of oral contraceptives or hormone replacement

Lung Cancer – Linked to ;
- Intake of high doses of beta carotene supplements (especially in smokers)
- Large intakes of red meat, processed meat, and total fat
- Low intake vegetables (non-starchy) and fruits
- Overweight and obesity
- Tobacco smoke, exposure to second hand smoke, and other carcinogens (asbestos, aluminum, coal-tar fumes, iron and steel founding pollutants)

Prostate Cancer – Linked to;
- Diets high in calcium, but low in lycopene and selenium
- Large intakes of processed meat
- Inadequate physical activity
- Advanced age (older than 40)
- Family history of prostate cancer
- Ethnicity (being African American)

Colorectal Cancer – Linked to;
- Large intake of red meats and processed meats
- Abdominal body fatness, overweight and obesity
- High intakes of alcoholic drinks
- Low intakes of foods high in fiber
- Inadequate physical activity
- Inflammatory bowel disease (Crohn's disease, ulcerative colitis)

- Age

Cancers of the Head and Neck Region and Esophagus – Linked to;
- Alcohol consumption
- Smoking
- Low intake of vegetables (non-starchy) and fruit

(adapted from; *Food, Nutrition, Physical Activity, and the Prevention of Cancer: a Global Perspective.*)

CHAPTER 9

QUESTIONS ABOUT NUTRITION AND CANCER

These are questions that cancer patients may ask.

Q. *What can I do to prepare for treatment?*

A. The best way to prepare for treatment is to ask many questions about possible side effects and expected dietary restrictions. It would also be a good idea to start preparing a lot of foods that can be easily thawed if unable to prepare meals, quick high protein snacks, ready to eat vegetables, and plenty of clear fluids. Some of the best foods to have readily available would include chicken noodle soup, crackers, gelatin, graham crackers, peanut butter, cottage cheese, and canned fruit. This would also be a great time to talk with family and friends so they can help prepare meals, pick up groceries, or provide encouragement during periods of poor appetite or tiredness.

Q. *Why did the doctor tell me not to lose weight during treatment?*

A. Cancer patients should not try to lose weight during treatment because certain treatment related side effects may lead to weakness, tiredness, dehydration, and malnutrition. Too much weight loss during treatment can promote the development of preventable side effects, reduce the immune response, or result in a negative treatment response. Also, weight lost during cancer treatment could result in a greater loss of muscle and not fat. It would be best to speak with the physician to determine when the best time to lose weight.

Q. *Should I avoid all sugar if I have cancer?*

A. Sugar is necessary for every cell in our body so that it can be used to produce energy to complete simple tasks such as movements and breathing. Even if all sugar sources (bread, milk, ice cream, rice, fruits, etc.) were eliminated from the diet, the body can make sugar from fat and protein. Too much sugar intake can cause a rise in insulin levels which may contribute to elevated hormone levels which could promote unwanted growth of cancer cells. While under treatment, the doctor may recommend a high calorie diet that includes foods high in sugar. After treatment, the physician or dietitian may encourage a reduction in the amount of simple sugars consumed such as candy, cookies, high-sugar sodas, and other processed desserts.

Q. Should I take vitamins during treatment?

A. Intake of a variety of foods should be first priority. It is expected that majority of the vitamins and minerals the body is provided with come from food. In situations where intake is not adequate, a multivitamin may be warranted. Individuals should discuss the use of a multivitamin with the attending physician because some minerals and nutrients can react with cancer treatments, medications, or other pharmacologic therapies.

Q. Do cancer patients only have to eat organic foods?

A. Eating organic is a matter of choice. There is no scientific proof that organic foods will reduce cancer risk, they can be beneficial for those individuals who have allergies to substances in processed foods. The small amount of additives used in the present food supply has not been directly linked to causing cancer.

Q. If I have low blood counts as a result of cancer treatment, what should I eat?

A. If white blood counts are very low, certain foods should be eliminated to limit exposure to bacteria or other harmful agents. Measures should be taken to make sure that all foods are thoroughly cooked, fruits and vegetables are rinsed well, and foods are kept at proper storage temperatures. Patients should also be encouraged to avoid raw and unpasteurized dairy products, foods from a deli, unpasteurized foods, public salad and food bars, and undercooked meats.

Q. Should I consume my usual diet after I complete treatment?

A. After cancer treatment, patients should start to follow the current recommendations for cancer prevention. This includes increasing fiber in the diet, consuming a variety of plant based foods, reducing sodium intake, avoiding processed meats, be physically active, and try to achieve a healthy weight.

Q. *What types of foods are good for fighting cancer?*

A. The best way to fight cancer is to include a variety of fruits and vegetables. The diet should include bright and darkly colored vegetables such as cabbage, spinach, broccoli, onions, mustard greens, and sweet potatoes. Fruit choices should include strawberries, blackberries, blueberries, cranberries, honeydew melon, red or black grapes, plums, and grapefruit. Whole grain and high fiber foods should be included as well as foods high in omega 3 fats such as salmon and tuna. Adequate water should also be consumed to maintain hydration.

CHAPTER 10

NUTRITION PROTOCOLS

GOALS OF NUTRITION THERAPY

Nutrition therapy is an important part of the overall treatment for the Cancer patient. Goals for nutrition therapy during treatment should also be established and reviewed with patients
Listed below are several goals:

- Prevent malnutrition
- Prevent wasting of muscles
- Tolerance of treatment
- Reduce effects and complications
- Maintain strength and energy
- Fight infection
- Help recovery and healing
- improve quality of life

It is important to be attentive to patient's comments regarding food preferences, intake, and dietary choices so that the patient can achieve success through the treatment phase. This is often the stage where friends and family may be needed for support and motivation to treat food like medication or fuel for the body.

What foods should be encouraged?
Before, during, and after cancer treatment healthy lifestyle and food choices should be encouraged.

Encourage (especially before and during treatment) clients to:
- increase their intake of fruits and vegetables high in antioxidants
- whole grain cereals/ breads/ pastas,
- peanut butter, fish, dried beans,

- cheese, and milk.
- Fluids such as water, 100% fruit juices, and clear soups or broths.

Discourage clients from:
- smoking,
- increasing alcohol intake,
- avoiding physical activity

Recommend foods that are of high nutritional value.
For example:
- cooked greens,
- baked sweet potatoes,
- baked fish such as salmon or tuna (small amounts throughout the day)
- Strawberries, oranges, and blueberries (high in antioxidants)

A) Focus on Cancer Prevention

The most recent recommendations for cancer prevention were developed by the World Cancer Research Foundation and the American Institute for Cancer Research

This report suggests that cancer prevention strategies should help individuals (9):
- ♣ Be as lean as possible without becoming underweight
- ♣ Be physically active for at least 30 minutes everyday
- ♣ Avoid sugary drinks. Limit consumption of energy-dense foods high in added sugar, or low in fiber, or high in fat.
- ♣ Eat more of a variety of vegetable, fruits, whole grains, and legumes such as beans.
- ♣ Limit consumption of red meats (such as beef, poor, and lamb) and avoid processed meats.

♣ If consumed at all, limit alcoholic drinks.
- Men – 2 drinks/day
- Women -1 drink/day
  - Drink = 12 ozs of normal strength beer
    = one 1.5 oz measure of spirits such as vodka or whisky
    = one small 5 oz glass of wine

♣ Limit consumption of salty foods and foods processed with salt (sodium).

♣ Don't use supplements to protect against cancer.

♣ It is best for mothers to breast feed exclusively for up to 6 months then add other liquids and foods.

♣ After treatment, cancer survivors should follow the recommendations for cancer prevention.

B) After Diagnosis and Before Treatment

After cancer is diagnosed, the next step is to develop a plan of action regarding treatment of the disease. In the African-American community, some receive the diagnosis of cancer and forgo treatment due to fear of complicated side effects of treatment or failure of treatment to eliminate the disease. It should be made clear to African-American patients that treatment affects individuals differently and factors such as age, previous medical history, stage of the disease, general health, nutritional status, and goals of therapy all play a role in the type of therapy suggested or received. The three main types of therapies that are currently used to treat cancer patients include surgery, chemotherapy, and radiation therapy. More recently biologic, hormonal, and immunotherapy have gained some attention. Depending on the type and stage of cancer, cancer therapies can be used individually or combined to offer the best possible outcome. All treatment options should be discussed openly and thoroughly. The discussions should also illustrate specific pros and cons of each treatment so that patients can feel secure with choosing a treatment method. Well informed individuals who feel supported will put forth the best effort to undergo treatment with confidence and an optimistic attitude.

After diagnosis and before starting treatment, a nutritional assessment should be conducted. Nutritional evaluation should focus on correcting any nutritional deficiencies and encourage build up of nutrient stores with in the body. Sometimes, newly diagnosed cancer patients, need to be given the opportunity to freely discuss their own views regarding their cancer diagnosis, food perceptions, present nutrition related complications, and treatment outcome perceptions before a nutritional plan of care can be established.

Once rapport has been established;

- special emphasis should be directed towards beneficial nutritional practices and controlling weight.
- Emphasis should be directed towards increasing fruit and vegetable intake and reducing intake of nutrient inadequate, high fat processed foods and meats.
- Clear instructions should be given to individuals who have lost significant amounts of weight so that they are able to maintain or gain weight until the start of treatment.
- Specific guidelines about weight maintenance also should be provided to individuals that have gained significant amounts of weight or considered overweight.

To increase the chance of successful dietary compliance, early nutritional intervention should take place before the patient starts treatment and continue throughout treatment and on into the post-treatment stage. Initial nutritional discussions should;
- review principles that stress on eating a balanced diet,
- reducing consumption of unhealthy fats, limiting refined sugar products,
- reducing or avoiding alcohol,
- and limiting salt.
- good sources of protein and
- hydrating fluids

Family members can become a valuable asset when encouraging patients to stock up on healthy foods that require little preparation or assistance with future meal planning while undergoing treatment.

C) During Treatment

Once patients start treatment, the goals of therapy should be clearly outlined and understood by the patient. The goals should be personalized, focus on the type of cancer being treated, and review options and recommendations for treatment. It is very important that healthcare providers who deal with cancer patients be proactive before treatment starts. Proactive communication will lead to effective screening, assessment, and provide proper treatment in a timely fashion.

Types of Cancer Treatment and Potential Side Effects

Cancer Treatment	How it Can Affect Eating	What Sometimes Happens: Side Effects
Surgery	Increases the need for good nutrition. May slow digestion. May lessen the ability of the mouth, throat, and stomach to work properly. Adequate nutrition helps wound-healing and recovery.	Before surgery, a high-protein, high-calorie diet may be prescribed if a patient is underweight or weak. After surgery, some patients may not be able to eat normally. Temporarily nutrients may be provided through a needle by vein (such as in <u>total parenteral nutrition</u>), or through a tube in the nose or stomach.

Radiation Therapy	As it damages cancer cells, it also may affect healthy cells and healthy parts of the body.	Treatment of head, neck, chest, or breast may cause: • Dry mouth • Sore mouth • Sore throat • Difficulty swallowing (<u>dysphagia</u>) • Change in taste of food • Dental problems • Increased phlegm Treatment of stomach or pelvis may cause: • Nausea and vomiting • Diarrhea • Cramps, bloating
Chemotherapy	As it destroys cancer cells, it also may affect the digestive system and the desire or ability to eat.	• Nausea and vomiting • Loss of appetite • Diarrhea • Constipation • Sore mouth or throat • Weight gain or loss • Change in taste of food
Biological Therapy (Immunotherapy)	As it stimulates your immune system to fight cancer cells, it can affect the desire or ability to eat.	• Nausea and vomiting • Diarrhea • Sore mouth • Severe weight loss • Dry mouth • Change in taste of food • Muscle aches, fatigue, fever
Hormonal Therapy	Some types can increase appetite and change how the body handles fluids.	• Changes in appetite • Fluid retention

Source: National Cancer Institute. <u>http://www.cancer.gov/cancertopics/eatinghints/page7/#F1</u>.

Dealing With Side Effects

While side effects are not always present during cancer treatment, any cancer patient will tell you that this is probably the most fearful and complex subject to understand. At the initial diagnosis of cancer, patients are so overwhelmed with being diagnosed with cancer that they usually do not understand what may happen during treatment. Sometimes educational status, lack of motivation, lack of family support, economic status, and poor patient to healthcare professional relationship all can play an instrumental part in how side effects are managed. All patients should be informed of the potential side effects and nutritional management strategies that can reduce the risk of having negative treatment experiences and developing of complications before starting treatment and again when starting treatment.

Symptom Management (7)

Symptoms	Tips for Management	Food Options
Anorexia or Early Satiety	• Eat small frequent, high cal/ high protein meals and snacks • Add protein or calories to favorite foods • Try light exercise • Eat meals and snacks in a pleasant atmosphere • Drink nutrient –dense liquids or supplements between meals to avoid feeling too full with meals	Cheese and crackers, cottage cheese and canned peaches, cream based soups, peanut butter and jelly sandwiches, vegetable dips, fruit smoothies
Constipation	• Increase fluid intake • Increase dietary fiber • Try prune juice • Increase physical activity • Try to have a set schedule for routine bowel movements	Oatmeal, bran flakes, high fiber cereals, wheat bread, prune juice, apples, broccoli, hot tea

Diarrhea	• Increase fluid intake • Limit/avoid insoluble fiber • Avoid greasy, fried, spicy, or very rich foods. • Eat small, frequent meals and snacks throughout the day. • Avoid alcohol and caffeine	Applesauce, oatmeal, bananas, plain crackers, broth based soups, baked potatoes, weak tea, plain toast, yogurt
Nausea / Vomiting	• Try small frequent feedings • Try room temperature or cold foods • Consume clear liquids between meals • Consume ice chips throughout the day • Avoid fried, greasy, or spicy foods • Avoid strong odors. • If vomiting is related to thick secretions, increase fluids to thin secretions, rinse and gargle with a mix of 1 Tbsp baking soda and 1 qt of water, and limit caffeine and very sweet beverages.	Saltine crackers, broth soups, plain gelatin, popsicles, plain toast, ginger ale, pretzels, apple or white grape juice
Weight Loss	• Consume small frequent, nutrient dense meals • Consume high calorie / high protein snacks like custard, cottage cheese and fruit, or peanut butter milkshakes • Eat more when feeling well • Consume oral nutritional supplements and milkshakes between meals • Add dry milk powder to milk and soups	Ice cream, peanut butter and jelly sandwich, vegetables with butter, grits and melted cheese, egg salad, meat casseroles, oral supplements

Weight Gain	• Consume low fat foods • Increase fruit and vegetable intake • Drink more water • Light to moderate exercise if approved by doctor	High fiber cereals, baked fish, salads, low-fat dressings, water, raw fruits, raw vegetables
Dry Mouth / Thick Saliva	• Increase fluid intake • Avoid alcohol containing mouthwashes or caffeine containing beverages • Rinse mouth with a solution of 1 Tbsp of baking soda mixed with 1 qt of water • Try sucking on lemon drops or consume tart foods • Consume foods that are soft and have a lot of moisture	Popsicles, water, broth based soups, lemon candies, watermelon, yogurt, cornbread soaked in milk
Sore Throat	• Consume soft foods that are moist • Avoid acidic, rough, spicy, and dry foods • Try consuming room temperature or cool foods • Increase fluid intake • Gargle with a solution of 1 Tbsp of baking soda mixed with water throughout the day	Grits, oatmeal, cottage cheese, angel hair pasta, canned peaches, baked fish, scrambled eggs, milkshakes, creamed soups, baked sweet potato, cooked squash
Taste Changes	• Rinse mouth with baking soda and water solution before and after eating • Use plastic utensils instead of metal utensils • Try consuming fish, tuna, or eggs instead of red meats • Try to consume fresh or frozen foods instead of cooked foods • Try adding lemon juice to foods/ oral supplements that taste too sweet	Ham salad, baked turkey, baked fish with lemon juice, mild cheese, Italian salad dressing, ginger ale, yogurt, cooked beans

Dysphagia	• Encourage speech therapy evaluation at onset of symptoms • Consume foods that are moist and soft; may require a full liquid or pureed diet • Eat small meals every 2 hours • Use oral supplements to supplement the diet if adequate calories or protein is not consumed • Thicken foods with gelatin, commercial food thickeners, or instant mashed potatoes per speech therapy recommendations	Milkshakes, soups, milk, peach or pear nectar, pudding, oral supplements
Pain	• Encourage small meals every 2 hours • Drink plenty of water and non-caffeinated beverages between meals • Try cold foods • Take pain meds as directed and manage routine bowel movements	Fruit juices, soups, noodles, toast, crackers, cooked vegetables

D) After Treatment

Upon completion of treatment, the nutritional plan of the cancer patient should be geared towards recovery. Depending on the type of cancer and the side effects experienced during treatment, the patient should;

- continue to monitor weight, prevent weight loss/gain,
- consume foods that promote healing, and
- continue to follow up with the physician and dietitian routinely.

It is advantageous for the nutrition professional to encourage African-American cancer survivors to obtain and maintain a healthy weight after treatment.

The American Cancer Society recommends that individuals who have completed treatment:

- Check with the doctor for any food or diet restrictions.
- Ask a dietitian to help create a nutritious, balanced eating plan
- Choose a variety of foods from all food groups. Try to eat at least 5-7 servings a day of fruits and vegetables, including citrus fruits, and dark-green and deep-yellow vegetables.
- Eat plenty of high fiber foods, such as whole grain breads and cereals
- Buy a new fruit, vegetable, low-fat food, or whole grain product each time you shop for groceries
- Decrease the amount of fat in your meals by baking or broiling foods
- Choose low-fat milk and dairy products
- Avoid salt-cured, smoked, and pickled foods
- Drink alcohol only occasionally
- If overweight, consider losing weight by reducing the amount of fat in your diet and increasing your activity. Check with the doctor before starting any exercise program.

The American Institute for Cancer Research guidelines are very similar but adds that cancer survivors avoid charred food and practice proper food storage and preparation.

CHAPTER 11

MEAL PLANNING

SAMPLE FOOD IDEAS

High Calorie	Low Calorie Low Fat	Low Fiber	High Fiber
Cream Cheese	Graham crackers	White bread	Oatmeal
Ice Cream	Apple	Pasta	Whole Wheat Bread
Fried Foods	Bananas	Corn Flakes	Whole Wheat Pasta
Coffee Creamer	Water	Biscuits	Fig Newton
Butter	Rice cakes	Pancakes	Granola
Whipped Cream	Gelatin	Pretzels	Bran
Heavy Cream	Plain popcorn	Gelatin	Corn
Dried fruit	Pickles	Pudding	Raisin Bran
Granola	Tomatoes	Plain rice	High fiber cereals
Pudding	Carrot sticks	Vanilla wafers	Beans/peas
Mayonnaise	Strawberries	Grits	Brown rice
Chocolate	Blueberries	Soda crackers	Popcorn
Gravy	Skim milk	Baked potato	Broccoli
Cheese Sauce	1% milk	Cucumbers	Potato Skins
Marshmallows	Low-fat mayo	Green Beans	Apple skin
Avocado	Low-fat cheese		
Muffins	Grilled or baked meats		
	Low-fat yogurt		

High Protein	Clear Liquid	Full Liquid
Tuna	Broths	Clear Liquids
Fish	(chicken, beef, vegetable)	Cheese soups
Poultry	Ice Chips	Eggnog
Beef	Apple Juice	Sherbet
Milk	Cranberry Juice	Drinkable yogurt
Pork	White Grape juice	Milk
Egg yolks	Ginger Ale	Milkshakes
Dry milk powder	Clear sodas	Vegetable juice
Half and Half	Gelatin	Tomato soups
Evaporated Milk	Popsicles	Soft Custard
Peanut butter	Weak Tea	Smooth Ice Cream
Beans	Sports Drinks	Fruit nectars
Cheese		Liquid supplements
Cottage cheese		Tea
Nuts		Strained cooked cereal
Yogurt		Coffee
Custard		

Sample Eating Schedule

Weight Gain	Weight Loss
8 am – Oatmeal with blueberries Condensed milk Scrambled egg Wheat Toast with jam and butter Coffee with cream Water	8 am Oatmeal with blueberries Skim or low-fat milk Boiled egg Wheat Toast Coffee Water
10 am Cottage cheese with fruit Water	10 am Rice cake or banana Water
12 am Grilled cheese sandwich Cream of Broccoli Soup Club crackers Mixed fruit cup and whipped topping Fruit Punch	12 pm Grilled chicken in Spinach Salad Vegetable soup Wheat crackers Green apple Light Lemonade
2 pm Homemade Ice Cream Milkshake Water	2 pm Mixed nuts or Low calorie smoothie Water
5 pm Baked fish Mashed potatoes with sour cream Carrots with butter Chocolate pudding Sweet Tea Water	5 pm Baked fish Brown rice pilaf Steamed broccoli Angel food cake Unsweet Tea Water
7 pm Yogurt with fruit or Peanut butter and jelly sandwich and Milk	7 pm Low fat Yogurt Water

CHAPTER 12

USEFUL TERMS

Anemia – low red blood cell count

Anorexia – The loss of appetite that may be a side effect of cancer treatment or caused by the cancer itself.

Antioxidants – Chemical compounds that hold back chemical reactions with oxygen.

Benign – not cancerous

Cachexia – a profound state of general poor health and malnutrition

Cancer – a group of diseases that causes cells in the body to grow out of control.

Carcinogen – A substance that enhances or helps cancer grow.

Chemotherapy – a type of cancer treatment using drugs to destroy cancer cells

Dysphagia – difficulty swallowing or eating.

Edema – swelling caused by excess fluid in body tissues.

Immune system – the complex system by which the body resists infection by germs, such as bacteria or viruses and rejects transplanted tissues or organs.

Immunotherapy – treatment to boost or restore the ability of the immune system to fight cancer, infections, and other diseases.

Leukemia – cancer of the blood or blood forming organs

Lymphoma – a cancer of the lymphatic system, a network of thin vessels and nodes throughout the body that helps to fight infection.

Malignant tumor – a mass of cancer cells that may invade surrounding tissues or spread (metastasize) to distant areas of the body.

Metastasize – the spread of cancer cells to one or more sites elsewhere in the body, by way of the lymph system or bloodstream.

Metabolize - the total of all chemical changes that take palace in a cell or an organism which may produce energy and basic materials needed for important life processes.

Mucositis – an inflammation of a mucus membrane

Neutropenia – a decrease in the number of neutrophils (white blood cells that respond quickly to infection) in the blood.

Nutritional Counseling - A process by which a health professional with special training in nutrition helps people make healthy food choices and form healthy eating habits.

Oncologist – a doctor with special training in the diagnosis of and treatment of cancer.

Palliative treatment – treatment that relieves symptoms, but is not expected to cure the disease.

Radiation therapy – a type of cancer treatment using high-energy rays to kill or shrink cancer cells which can external or internal.

Registered dietitian – the expert in the area of foods and diet that has at least a bachelor's degree and has passed a national competency exam.

Remission – complete or partial disappearance of the signs and symptoms of cancer in response to treatment and is considered as the period during which the disease is under control.

Screening – to check for disease when there are no symptoms

Terminal – generally understood to mean that the cancer is no longer considered curable, and the patient is dying.

Tumor – an abnormal lump or mass of tissue.

Xerostomia – dry mouth due to lack of saliva

CHAPTER 13

RESOURCES FOR NUTRITION AND CANCER

Books

Informed Decisions: The Complete Book of Cancer Diagnosis, Treatment, and Recovery edited by Harmon J. Eyre, M.D., Diane Partie Lange, and Lois Morris (American Cancer Society)

Good For You! Reducing Your Risk of Developing Cancer. (American Cancer Society).

The Cancer Survival Cookbook by D. Weihofen

Eating Well Through Cancer: Easy Recipes and Recommendations During and After Treatment by Holly Clegg

Eating Well, Staying Well: During and After Cancer by Abby Bloch. (American Cancer Society)

Brochures

Eating Hints for Cancer Patients: Before, During, and After Treatment. National Cancer Institute (NCI) – http://www.cancer.gov/cancertopics/eatinghints

Nutrition of the Cancer Patient. American Institute of Cancer Research

Web Resources

American Cancer Society- http://www.cancer.org/docroot/home/index.asp

American Institute for Cancer Research - http://www.aicr.org/site/PageServer

Caring 4 Cancer – Nutrition Section - http://www.caring4cancer.com

Food, Nutrition, Physical Activity, and the Prevention of Cancer: a Global Perspective – Online - http://www.dietandcancerreport.org

National Cancer Institute - http://www.cancer.gov

Oncolink - http://www.oncolink.com

Herbs and Supplements References

The National Center for Complementary and Alternative Therapy (NCCAM) - http://nccam.nih.gov/

The Office of Dietary Supplements - http://dietary-supplements.info.nih.gov/

American Botanical Council - http://www.herbalgram.org/

Dietary Supplements - Warnings and Safety - http://www.cfsan.fda.gov/~dms/ds-warn.html

PDR Natural Medicine - http://www.pdrhealth.com/drugs/altmed/altmed-a-z.aspx

Helpful Organizations

General Cancers
Leukemia and Lymphoma Society – www.leukemia.org
Livestrong: Lance Armstrong Foundation – www.livestrong.org

Breast Cancer
Susan G. Komen for the Cure – ww5.komen.org
Breast Cancer Network of Strength – www.networkofstrength.org

Lung Cancer
Alliance for Lung Cancer Advocacy, Support and Education (ALCASE)- www.alcase.org
Lung Cancer Online – www.lungcanceronline.org

Colon Cancer
Colon Cancer Alliance – www.ccalliance.org

Head and Neck Cancers
Supporting People with Oral and Head and Neck Cancer – www.spohnc.org

Pancreatic Cancer
The Pancreatic Cancer Action Network (PANCAN) – www.pancan.org

Prostate Cancer
Prostate Cancer Foundation – www.prostatecancerfoundation.org
US-TOO Prostate Cancer Education & Support – www.ustoo.com

PATIENT INFORMATION

The material in this section is to be used as a handout for the patients

TIPS TO REDUCE NAUSEA AND VOMITING

- Consume small frequent meals (around 6-8 per day)

- Suck on Ice chips

- Drink clear carbonated beverages, broths, lemonade, ginger ale, or tea between meals

- Nibble on salty crackers, pretzels, low fat potato chips, or toast

- Try cold foods such as popsicles, sherbet, and yogurt

- land foods such as baked chicken, baked potatoes, angel food cake, and hot cereals

- Avoid food with strong smells

- Do not take anti-nausea medicines on an empty stomach

- Sit up during all meals and snacks and for at least 45 minutes after eating

- Refrain from consuming greasy, spicy and fried or fatty foods

REFERENCES

U.S. Cancer Statistics Working Group. *United States Cancer Statistics: 2004 Incidence and Mortality.* Atlanta: U.S. Department of Health and Human Services, Centers for Disease Control and Prevention *and* National Cancer Institute; 2007.

Matthews A.K, Sellergren S.A., Manfredi C., Williams M. Factors Influencing Medical Information Seeking Among African American Cancer Patients. *J Health Comm.* May 2002:7;205-219.

American Cancer Society. Cancer Facts & Figures for African Americans 2007-2008. Atlanta: American Cancer Society; 2007. Available at: http://www.cancer.org/downloads/STT/CAFF2007AAacspdf2007.pdf. Accessed on: May 29, 2008.

Clegg H, Miletello G. Eating Well Through Cancer. Memphis, Tenn: Wimmer Cookbooks; 2001.

Trujillo E, Nebeling L. Changes in Carbohydrate, Lipid, and Protein Metabolism in Cancer. In McCallum PD, Polisena CG, eds. *The Clinical Guide to Oncology Nutrition.* Chicago, IL: American Dietetic Association; 2000:17-25.

World Cancer Research Fund / American Institute for Cancer Research. Food, Nutrition, Physical Activity, and the Prevention of Cancer: a Global Perspective. Washington DC: AICR, 2007. Available at http://www.dietandcancerreport.org. Accessed on July 5, 2009.

Schattner M, Shike M. Nutrition support of the patient with cancer. In: Shils M, Shike M, Ross A, Caballero B, Cousins R. *Modern Nutrition in Health and Disease.* 10ed. 1290-1313.

Nutrition in Cancer Care. Nutrition Therapy Overview. National Cancer Institute Website. Available at: http://www.cancer.gov/cancertopics/pdq/supportivecare /nutrition/Patient/page4. Accessed on July 1, 2007.

Appendix A. Tips for Managing Nutrition Impact Symptoms. In: Elliot L, Molseed L, McCallum P, and Grant B. *The Clinical Guide to Oncology Nutrition*. 2nd ed. Chicago, IL: American Dietetic Association;2006:241-245.

Bloch AS. Cancer. In: Glottschlich MM, Matarese LD, Shronts EP, eds. Nutrition Support in Dietetics Core Curriculum. 2nd ed. Silver Spring, MD: *American Society for Parenteral and Enteral Nutrition*; 1993: 213-226.

Kogut, V and Luthringer S, eds. Nutritional Issues in Cancer Care. Pittsburg, PA: Oncology Nursing Society;2005:104-138.

In: Elliot L, Molseed L, McCallum P, and Grant B. *The Clinical Guide to Oncology Nutrition*. 2nd ed. Chicago, IL: American Dietetic Association;2006:29-31.

World Cancer Research Fund / American Institute for Cancer Research. Food, Nutrition, Physical Activity, and the Prevention of Cancer: a Global Perspective. Washington DC: AICR, 2007. Available at http://www.dietandcancerreport.org. Accessed on July 5, 2009.

In: Elliot L, Molseed L, McCallum P, and Grant B. *The Clinical Guide to Oncology Nutrition*. 2nd ed. Chicago, IL: American Dietetic Association;2006:187.

Rock CL, Doyle C, Demark-Wahnefried W, et al. Nutrition and physical activity guidelines for cancer survivors. *CA Cancer JClin*. 2012;62 (4)243-274.

Fox N. Using nutrition intervention to resolve nutrition impact symptoms and save healthcare dollars. *Oncology Nutrition Connection*. 2013;21(1); 15-17.

Elliott L, Levin R, McIver J. Complete Resource Kit for Oncology Nutrition. AND Publications; 2012

Brown CG. A Guide to Oncology Symptom Management. Pittsburgh, PA: Oncology Nursing Society, 2010.

Bovell-Benjamin A, Dawkins N, Pace R, Shaikany JM. Dietary consumption practices and cancer risk in African Americans in the rural south. *J Health Care Poor Underserved*. 2010:21(3);57-75.

HYPERTENSION

PART - 3

THE AFRICAN-AMERICAN HYPERTENSION OVERVIEW

INTRODUCTION

Hypertension, commonly termed high blood pressure, is a major public health problem not just in the United States of America, but in countries world-wide. Due to the asymptomatic nature of this disease it may go undetected and undiagnosed for many years in all populations at risk.

More than any other race or ethnic group, African Americans are at high risk for developing hypertension. In fact, the prevalence of high blood pressure among African Americans is among the highest in the world. The rates of hypertension in Hispanic Americans, Caucasians, and Native Americans are very similar (ranging from 24% to 27%). The rate is much lower in Asian Pacific Islanders (9.7% in men and 8.4% in women). There seems to be no definitive reason for this obvious difference in the incidence of the disease between other races and ethnic groups. The 'Well-Connected Report' March 2002, which was edited by Harvey Simon, MD, Editor-in-Chief, Associate Professor of Medicine, Harvard Medical School; reported that a number of theories have surfaced addressing the reasons for this difference. These theories suggest that;

- "Some studies have indicated that African Americans may have lower levels of nitric oxide and higher levels of a peptide called endothelin-1 (ET-1) than Caucasians. (Nitric oxide keeps blood vessels flexible and open and ET-1 narrows blood vessels.)
- African Americans have a higher risk for an impaired response to angiotensin (Ang II), which is a peptide important in regulating salt and water balances. (African Americans are more likely to be salt-sensitive than other groups.)
- income disparities and dietary issues may explain many of the differences in blood pressure rates observed between ethnic groups.

In any case, inadequately controlled hypertension is the major factor for the higher mortality rate from heart disease among African Americans".

Hypertension, (high blood pressure) which is sometimes called the silent killer due to the frequent lack of symptoms or discomfort, is a major risk factor for cardiovascular, disease, stroke, and kidney disease. High blood cholesterol is also a risk factor for heart disease. Fortunately both high blood pressure and high blood cholesterol can be controlled in part by making some simple changes in what you eat. Cutting back on salt and sodium can help lower blood pressure.

CHAPTER 14

QUESTIONS ABOUT NUTRITION AND HIGH BLOOD PRESSURE

Q. *What is blood pressure?*

A. It is the force or push of blood as it flows through the blood vessels.

Q. *What is high blood pressure?*

A. Blood pressure normally goes up and down in response to body demands and activities. When your numbers are consistently above 139/89mm Hg *(systolic/diastolic) you are experiencing high blood pressure or hypertension (medical term for high blood pressure). Excellent blood pressure would be less than 120/80mm Hg.

- **Systolic**: the systolic pressure is the first and usually the higher number, and it is the measurement of the force that blood exerts on the artery walls as the heart contracts to pump out the blood.

- **Diastolic**: the diastolic pressure is the second and usually the lower number, and it is the measurement of the force as the heart relaxes to allow the blood to flow into the heart.

- **mm Hg**: Blood pressure is measured in millimeters of mercury.

Q. *What are some facts about high blood pressure?*

A. One out of every four Americans has high blood pressure. One out of every three African Americans has high blood pressure. High blood pressure has no clear symptoms. A person can have high blood pressure and not know it. High blood pressure cannot be cured, but it can be controlled.

Hypertension is classified in two ways;

- **Essential or primary hypertension**: Ninety five percent (95%) of all persons diagnosed will be in this group. Essential hypertension is of unknown etiology, but is positively influenced by modified behavioral patterns and dietary intake.

- **Secondary hypertension**: The reminding five percent (5%) of all persons diagnosed will be in this group. Secondary hypertension is less common, and is usually present because of some other medical condition such as renal, endocrine or neurologic disorders.

Q. *Does what we eat affect blood pressure?*
A. Yes. Eating foods that are very high in salt can increase the blood pressure in people who are sensitive to it.

Q. *What do we know about weight and high blood pressure?*

High blood pressure is more common in overweight people. As a person gains weight, blood pressure tends to rise; when a person loses weight, blood pressure often goes down.

About one-third of patients with high-blood pressure are overweight.

Even if the patient is moderately obese, the risk of developing hypertension will be twice that of a patient within normal parameters.

Q. *Will maintaining a healthy weight prevent high blood pressure?*
A. No one knows for sure, but maintaining a healthy weight may reduce the risk of getting high blood pressure. In fact blood pressure rises as body weight increases.
- There are two methods used to determine if one is of healthy weight; the BMI (Body Mass Index) and Waist circumference.
- 'BMI' measures the weight relative to the height, but may over or under estimate body fat.
- 'Waist measurement' checks abdominal fat. A waist measurement of more than 35 inches in women and more than 40 inches in men is considered high – increases the risk of hypertension.

Q. *What is the best way to lose weight?*

A. The best way to lose weight is to eat a variety of foods each day; reduce the fat and sugar content of your diet by replacing desserts and snacks with fruits and vegetables; and include some type of exercise, like a vigorous walk, in your daily routine. A BMI less than 25 is ideal, and supports a heart healthy lifestyle.
- BMI of 25 to 29.9 -   Overweight
- BMI of 30 or greater - Obese

Q. *How much sodium is too much?*

A. A reasonable amount of sodium in the diet of the average person is 2 grams (2000 mg) daily, which is equal to the amount of sodium found in 1 teaspoon of salt. Most Americans eat 2 to 4 times more sodium than they need by salting their foods and eating foods high in sodium.
- **FYI: Table Salt**
  Table salt is a mixture of two substances – sodium and chloride. There is 40 percent sodium and 60 percent chloride in table salt. One teaspoon of salt = 2000 mg. sodium.

Q. *What about using salt substitutes?*

A. If you want to use salt substitutes, choose those that do not contain potassium chloride (KCl). There are several brands available. Ask your doctor before you make a decision to try salt substitutes.

Q. *Are there specific diets for people with high blood pressure?*

A. No, but doctors and dietitians often provide calorie and sodium controlled diets, tailored to each person's medical condition, food preferences and lifestyle. Dietitians and Nutritionists can also give tips on how to shop for appropriate foods, and how to prepare tasty meals with little or no salt.

The DASH (Dietary Approach to Stop Hypertension) Diet is now often recommended as the principle diet therapy in managing blood pressure;
- Avoid saturated fat
- Select monounsaturated oils, such as olive or canola oils
- Choose whole grains over white flour or pasta products

- Choose fresh fruits and vegetables every day,
- Include nuts, seeds or legumes (dried beans & peas) daily.
- Choose modest amounts of protein
- Fish: especially oily fish containing omega-3 fatty acids.
- Soy: in combination with fiber-rich foods

Supplements may have specific benefits should be presented to the patient.

Changing eating habits can be a fun challenge, but it takes time. Friends and family of patients can help by being supportive in an effort to help them make permanent changes towards a healthier lifestyle.

Source: adapted from the Manual of Clinical Dietetics – 7th Edition, 2007
Source: adapted from NIH publications No.-2024, September 1987; and 88-1459 September 198

CHAPTER 15

NUTRITION ASSESSMENT - HYPERTENSION

The assessment, diagnosis and treatment of patients with hypertension are a team effort. The health care team, which is comprised of the physician, nurse, dietitian, pharmacist and other health professionals, determines the medical and the nutritional protocol to be followed, to maintain a healthy lifestyle. This process starts with a confirmed diagnosis of hypertension which is determined by measuring blood pressure.

The procedural steps:

A. The physical examination will include blood pressure measurements
   - The measurement will be taken using a sphygmomanometer, while the patient is seated upright.
   - The health care worker taking the blood pressure listens through a stethoscope.
   - The systolic and the diastolic blood pressures are recorded in the medical chart.
   - The diagnosis of hypertension is determined by at least two elevated blood pressure readings on two or more occasions. (Considered high; when the readings are greater than 139/89 mm Hg)

False 'low' pressure reading can be caused by:
   - Recent exercise
   - Not smoking – after heavy, long-term smoking

False 'high' pressure reading can be caused by:
   - An arm cuff place too tightly, or one that is too small
   - Talking during the test
   - Consumption of coffee (caffeine containing beverages) before testing

    -   Stress or tension

B. The nutritional assessment then continues with;
- Health history
- Medication history
- Personal history
- Diet history

C. Additional test also help to classify the type of hypertension manifested in the patient. These tests may include, but are not limited to:
- Blood test and urinalysis
- An electrocardiogram (ECG)
- A stress test

The findings are them evaluated and the relevance to the patient's nutritional condition discussed. The appropriate treatment is then designed and implemented by the health care team.

CHAPTER 16

NUTRITION PROTOCOLS

Hypertension or high blood pressure cannot be cured in most cases, but it can be effectively managed, therefore providing a better quality of life for the patient.

The medical therapy for this disease requires lifestyle changes involving diet and medication.

The nutrition therapy plan for the hypertensive patient is best accomplished using the specialized skills of a registered dietitian (RD). When the RD is unavailable the dietary guidance of the patient may fall on other member of the health care team. The following nutrition therapy plans should be used to initiate and or monitor the diet until the RD is able to do so.

The National High Blood Pressure Education Program (NHBPEP) recommends a diet that contains 2000-2400 mg. sodium (approximately 1 teaspoon salt), for patients with hypertension. The DASH (Dietary Approach to Stop Hypertension) –sodium study however, showed greater results with a diet that had a sodium content of 1500 mg. daily. .

The DASH Diet is now often recommended as the principle diet therapy in managing blood pressure. It is recommended that patients:
- *Avoid saturated fat*
- *When choosing fat, select monounsaturated oils, such as olive or canola oils*
- *Choose whole grains over white flour or pasta products*
- *Choose fresh fruits and vegetables every day, especially those that are rich in fiber; (lowers blood pressure) and potassium; and Vitamin C; (boost the effects of calcium-channel blocking drugs).*
- *Include nuts, seeds or legumes (dried beans & peas) daily.*

- *Choose modest amounts of protein*
  - *Fish: especially oily fish is beneficial because they contain omega-3 fatty acids.*
  - *Soy: in combination with fiber-rich foods or supplements may have specific benefits should be presented to the patient.*

Serving sizes used with the High Blood Pressure Diet - DASH

Diet based on 2000 Kcal, and 1500 mg Sodium daily.

Grain	7 – 8 servings
Vegetables	4 – 5 servings
Fruits	4 – 5 servings
Low fat or Fat-free Dairy	2 – 3 servings
Meats, poultry & Fish	2 or less servings
Nuts, seeds & Dry beans	4 – 5 servings per week
Fats & Oils	2 – 3 servings
Sweets	5 servings per week

To assist the patient with adhering to the low sodium diet lifestyle, a list of special considerations has been generated and should be used as the steps to success when teaching or counseling.

**The following guide may be copied
and used as a handout.**

STEPS TO SUCCESS
Low-Sodium Diet Lifestyle.

Read Food Labels	Check the nutrition facts label for sodium content.
Limit Consumption of High-Sodium Processed Food	Includes pre-packaged, frozen and canned foods
Remove the Salt Shaker from the Table	Refrain from purchasing salt at the grocery
Add Flavor with Herbs And Spices	These all add flavor without adding sodium
Beware of Salt Substitutes	Read the labels, and if taking blood pressure medication, consult your physician before using the salt substitute.
Maintain a Healthy	Regular exercise is important in helping to lose
Body Weight and	weight and maintain weight loss. It also keeps
Exercise Regularly	blood pressure down.
Alcohol in Moderation	Consume no more than one ounce per day
Eat Potassium-rich Foods	Works in concert with sodium to regulate blood pressure.

ONE DAY SAMPLE MENU: approximately 1500 mg sodium

BREAKFAST:

½ c.	orange juice
1 c.	Oatmeal
1 c.	Skim (or fat-free) milk
2 sl.	Whole wheat toast with low-sodium margarine
1 med.	Banana
1 c.	decaffeinated coffee

LUNCH:

½ c.	fruit cup (natural juices)
3 ozs.	grilled Chicken breast
½ c.	grilled Zucchini
½ c.	Pasta salad with low-sodium dressing
1 sl.	Italian Bread
1 tsp.	Low-sodium margarine
1 c.	skim (fat-free) milk

DINNER:

4 ozs.	Halibut or Trout (broiled)
½ c.	Broccoli
2	Boiled potatoes with parsley
1	whole wheat roll
1 tsp.	Low-sodium margarine
1 c.	mixed lettuce greens with oil & vinegar dressing
½ c.	sherbet
1 c.	decaffeinated coffee

SUBSTITUTION SUGGESTIONS:

RATHER THAN:	WHY NOT TRY:
1 cup butter	7/8 cup vegetable oil, or 1 cup tub margarine, or 1 cup (2 sticks) margarine
1 cup heavy cream	1 cup evaporated skim milk
1 medium whole egg	2 egg whites
2 egg yolks	1 whole egg
1 cup whole milk	1 cup skim milk
1 cup sour cream	1 cup plain low-fat yogurt
1 ounce baking chocolate	3 Tbsp. Cocoa powder blended with 1 Tbsp. Vegetable oil
1 cup mayonnaise	1 cup low calorie salad dressing

CHAPTER 17

DIET – DRUG INTERACTIONS

Food and Drugs (or medication) interacts in various and complex ways. Foods eaten may have an effect on the medications given, causing the medication to become more powerful causing can interference with the body's ability to absorb nutrients.

It is important to understand the interaction of food with the prescribed medication because some clients may experience loss of appetite, dry mouth, weight gain, weakness, nausea, diarrhea or constipation.

GENERAL INFORMATION:

If the patient has been prescribed a hypertensive medication, make sure that they are aware that;
- Medication is taken at the same time every day
- Follow the directions regarding taking the medication with or without food
- Do not eat salty foods or add salt to the food
- Consume a diet with adequate calories
- Eat fruits and vegetables, especially those high in potassium, daily. Many hypertensive medications remove potassium from the body.

When a diuretic (fluid pill) has been prescribed, suggested that;
- Take the medication at the same time every day
- If the diuretic upsets the stomach, take it with food
- Avoid high –sodium (salt) foods
- Eat fruits and vegetables, especially those high in potassium, daily.
- Avoid using potassium-containing salt substitute
- Avoid sodium-containing antacids
- Drink a low-fat milk/milk product daily to help increase calcium and vitamin D, reducing the risk of osteoporosis

There are many medications prescribed to help lower blood pressure. With new medications becoming available constantly, a listing of the names of the drugs available in the marketplace would become incomplete almost daily. All medications fall into nine main categories however, and each category works in various ways.

Many patients will be taking two or more types of prescribed medication to bring their pressure down to a health level.

CATEGORY OF MEDICATION	WHAT DOES IT DO?
**Diuretics	Called 'water pills'. They flush excess water and sodium through the kidneys, and remove them from the body in the urine.
Beta-blockers	Makes the heart beat less often and with less force by reducing the nerve impulses sent to the heart and blood vessels. The blood pressure drops, and the heart works less hard.
Angiotensin converting enzymes inhibitors	Prevents the formation of a hormone called angiotensin11, which normally causes blood vessels to narrow. The blood vessels relax, and pressure goes down.
Angiotensin antagonists	These protect blood vessels from angiotensin11. As a result the blood vessels open wider, and pressure goes down.
Calcium channel blockers	Keep calcium from entering the muscle cells of the heart and blood vessels. Blood vessels, allowing blood to pass more easily.
Alpha-blockers	Allows blood to pass more easily through the blood vessels by reducing nerve impulses.

Alpha-beta-blockers	Combines the function of the alpha-blocker and the beta-blocker: reduces nerve impulses to blood vessels and also slows the heartbeat.
Nervous system inhibitors	These relax blood vessels by controlling nerve impulses.
Vasodilators	These directly open blood vessels by relaxing the muscle in the vessel walls

Source: adapted from *Manage your Blood Pressure Drugs*

WEB RESOURCES

www.fda.gov/downloads/drugs
www.eatright.org/pubic/content
www.aafp.org/afp/2008
www.heart.org/medication-interactions

ADDITIONAL INFORMATION:

**For African Americans.
- Diuretics; respond well to these drugs
- ACE inhibitors are effective and also protect the kidneys
- Calcium-channel blockers are often, they are very expensive

Patients with Diabetes:
- need to control their blood pressure to 130/85 mm Hg or lower to protect the heart and help prevent other complications common to both diseases.
- ACE inhibitors are the first
- Combinations are required to achieve blood pressure goals

Patients with Obesity:

- Losing weight is critical,
- Some newer and effective weight-loss agents, such as sibutramine (Meridia), may actually raise blood pressure.
- ACE inhibitors and angiotensin receptor blockers may be helpful

REMEMBER:

Recommend to all patients to;

- Take the medication as prescribed
- Some over-the-counter drugs can raise your blood pressure because of the high sodium content. Make a habit of carefully reading the labels of all over-the-counter drugs. Check for the sodium content. Be cautious of;
  - Arthritis medications
  - Pain medications
  - Dietary supplements (ephedra, ma-huang, bitter orange)
  - Antacids; containing more than 5 milligrams

HELPFUL - TIPS

To help patients remember to take their medication, suggest that they:

- *Put the blood pressure medication on the night stand next to the bead*
- *Put the medication in a weekly pillbox*
- *Ask a child or grandchild to remind you daily*
- *Put a reminder note in a visible place; refrigerator, mirror, bedroom door*
- *Set up a buddy system with someone with hypertension*

OTHER NUTRIENTS AND BLOOD PRESSURE

FIBER
The benefits of a high-fiber diet are dramatic in persons with high blood pressure. An emphasis on fresh vegetables, fruits, and whole grain cereals, breads, and pastas are important, since these are high fiber foods. Fiber helps to modulate the amount of salt consumed, therefore helping to prevent hypertension and the metabolic results of hypertension: kidney and heart disease.

POTASSIUM
Dietary potassium may play a role in decreasing blood pressure. Increasing potassium in the diet may protect against hypertension in people who are sensitive to high levels of sodium. The American Heart Association recommends a sodium-to-potassium ratio of one-to-one, or equal amounts of sodium and potassium. However, taking potassium supplements is generally not recommended for people with high blood pressure. Instead, a variety of potassium-rich foods should be eaten daily.

ALCOHOL
Ten percent of hypertension cases are caused by alcohol abuse. Moderate drinking however, (one or two drinks a day) has benefits for the heart and may even protect against some types of stroke; but even low or moderate drinking may increase the risk for hypertension in African Americans. Red wine specifically may have chemicals that benefit blood pressure. (Red grape juice may have the same advantages)

CAFFEINE
Caffeine causes a temporary increase in blood pressure. Regular, heavy coffee consumption (an average of 5 cups per day) will boost blood pressure, and may be harmful in people with hypertension and may even increase their risk for stroke.

HERBAL SUPPLEMENTS

Herbal supplements are often used to treat hypertension however, they have serious side effects if taken in large doses. It is recommended that these herbs be used only under the supervision of a physician.

- **Fish Oil / Omega-3 Fatty Acids** – Some studies show small reductions in blood pressure; there are some limitations in role of managing high blood pressure without salt reduction, weight loss, exercise, and anti-hypertensive drug therapy.
- **Coenzyme Q 10** – preliminary research suggests that coenzyme Q10 can cause a small decrease in blood pressure, but long-term research is needed to strengthen this recommendation.
- **Coleus forskohlii** -Lowers blood pressure and improves heart function.
- **Hawthorne** -Has the ability to dilate coronary blood vessels, which helps lower blood pressure.
- **Mistletoe** -Not as potent as Rauwolfia but well tolerated and nontoxic in normal doses.
- **Rauwolfia** -This is considered the most powerful hypotensive botanical. Only a small dose is required to achieve results and to avoid side effects. Nasal congestion is the most common side effect.

Source: *Cardiology Channel; Hypertension*
Source: *Natural Standard Herb & Supplement Handbook: The Clinical Bottom Line By E. Basch and C. Ulbricht*

CHAPTER 18

HERBS & HERBAL SHAKERS

Most Americans, especially African Americans and the Elderly are sensitive to salt and sodium, and usually use more of these substances than is needed in food preparation.

Salt substitutes are acceptable, if approved by the doctor, but better yet, try the following seasonings with your favorite foods. These herbal seasonings also make a great flavor booster when combined and used as an herbal shaker.

Spice it up !!!

Herbs & Spices	Uses
Allspice	Lean meats, stews, Tomatoes, applesauce, Gravies, peaches
Basil	Lean meat, Fish, Lamb, Salads, Soups, Sauces
Bay Leaves	Lean meat, Stews, Poultry, Soups, Tomatoes
Caraway Seeds	Lean meats, Stews, Salads Breads, Noodles, Soups
Chives	Salads, Sauces,

	Soups, Lean meat, Cabbage, noodles
Cinnamon	Salads, Vegetables, Fruits, Breads, Snacks, Piecrust
Chili Powder	Fish, Soups, Salads
Curry Powder	Lean meats, Veal, Chicken Fish, tomatoes, Soup
Cloves	Soups, Ham, Salads,
Dill (weed & seed)	Soups, Beef, Lamb, Chicken, Fish, vegetables, Salads
Garlic	Lean meat, Fish, Soups, Salads, Vegetables, Pork
Ginger	Lean meats, Salads, Chicken, Fruits, Beverages
Lemon/Lime Juice	Fish, Salads, Vegetables
Mace	Hot breads, Apples, Veal, Lamb, Vegetables, Salads
Marjoram	Beef, Fish, Chicken, Soups, Salads, Vegetables
Nutmeg	Fruits, Lean meats, Veal, Fish, Vegetables, Potatoes

Oregano	Soups, Salads, Tomatoes, Lean ground meat, Sauces
Paprika	Lean meats, Fish, Soups, Salads, Sauces, Vegetables
Parsley	Lean meats, Fish, Soups, Sauces
Rosemary	Chicken, Veal, Pork, Lean meat Potatoes, Sauces
Sage	Lean meats, Stews, Vegetables, Biscuits, Onions
Thyme	Lean meats, Veal, Pork, Salads, Soups, Vegetables, Tomatoes

Experiment with these herbs and spices to spice up low-sodium or salt free meals!!

HERBAL SHAKERS:

Mixtures and shakers can be purchased at the supermarket but here are a few which are proven 'flavor boosters". They can be used instead of salt on many types of foods.

**For a shaker use a clean glass jar with a plastic screw top; store in a dry place.

Shaker #1		Shaker #2	
1 ½ tsp.	Thyme	1 tsp.	Celery Seed
1 ½ tsp.	Sage	2 ½ tsp.	Marjoram
2 tsp.	Rosemary	1 ½ tsp.	Savory
2 tsp.	Marjoram	1 ½ tsp.	Thyme
2 ½ tsp.	Savory	1 ½ tsp.	Basil

Shaker #3		Shaker #4	
2 ½ tsp.	Paprika	2 tbsp.	Crushed Savory
2 ½ tsp.	Garlic Powder	1 tbsp.	Dry Mustard
2 ½ tsp.	Dry Mustard	1 ½ tsp.	Onion Powder
5 tsp.	Onion Powder	1 ½ tsp.	Curry Powder
½ tsp.	Pepper	1 ¼ tsp	White Pepper
¼ tsp.	Celery Seed	1 tsp.	Ground Cumin
½ tsp.	Parsley Flakes	½ tsp.	Garlic Powder

Source: adapted from "Recipes for the Heart"

Shaker #5

2 tbsp.	Dillweed or Crushed Basil Leaves
1 tsp.	Crushed Oregano Leaves
2 tbsp.	Onion Powder
1 tsp.	Celery Seed
¼ tsp.	Dried Grated Lemon Peel

All Purpose Herbal Shaker

Shaker #6

5 tsp.	Onion Powder
2 ½ tsp.	Garlic Powder
2 ½ tsp.	Paprika
2 ½ tsp.	Dry Mustard
1 ½ tsp.	Thyme Leaves
½ tsp.	White Pepper
¼ tsp.	Celery Seeds

CHAPTER 19

FOOD LABELS

Sodium (salt) is found naturally in food. Processed foods however have addition sodium compounds incorporated in the product as a necessary function of processing. Processed foods (canned and in some cases frozen foods), have high levels of sodium per serving. The importance of reading the food label on all foods products purchased for consumption must be stressed to all patients especially African American patients.

Always read the label of any food product purchased and select only foods that are identified as being low in sodium.

Certain compounds that provide sodium to the diet are listed below. These products should be avoided.

Monosodium Glutamate (MSG):   use in restaurants and hotel cooking. Found in many packaged, canned and frozen foods.

Sodium Benzoate: used as a preservative in certain condiments, like relishes, sauces and salad dressings.

Sodium Propionate: used in pasteurized cheese and in some breads

Disodium Phosphate   used in some quick-cooking cereals and Process cheeses

| Sodium Hydroxide | used in food processing to softer and loosen skins of ripe olives and certain fruits and vegetables. |
| Sodium Alginate | used in many chocolate milks and ice Creams to make a smooth mixture. |

Source: *adopted from Shaking your salt Habit*

THE LABEL LINGO

Cooking with salt and salt containing products may seem so natural that it is done with out much notice. Patients that are salt sensitive must stop, and think before cooking. Products that are low-sodium or sodium-free must be used in place of high sodium processed foods.

What do the terms 'sodium-free', 'low-sodium' or even 'salt-free' really mean when they appear on the nutritional label?

LABEL TERMS	MEANING
Sodium free	Less then 5 milligrams sodium per serving
Very low sodium	35 milligrams or less sodium per serving
Reduced or Less sodium	At least 25% less sodium*
Light in sodium	50% less sodium* restricted to foods with more than 40 Kcalories per serving or more than 3 grams fat per serving.
Low sodium	140 milligrams or less sodium per serving

Low sodium meal	140 milligrams or less sodium per 100 grams
Salt free	Less than 5 milligrams sodium per serving
Unsalted or no added salt	No salt added during processing; does not necessarily mean sodium free

* as compared with a standard serving size of the traditional food

SODIUM CONTENT OF POPULAR FOODS

FOOD	SERVING	SODIUM (MG)
Milk Group		
Skim Milk	1 cup	122
Buttermilk	1 cup	257
Yogurt – low fat	1 cup	159
Ice Cream- vanilla	1 cup	112
Cheeses		
Swiss	1 oz.	74
Cheddar	1 oz	176
Processed American	1 oz.	406
Parmesan	1 oz.	454
Bread & Cereal Group		
White Bread	1 slice	114
Wheat Bread	1 slice	132
Cereals		
Grits, regular	¾ cup	0
Grits, instant	¾ cup	354
Oatmeal, regular	¾ cup	1
Oatmeal, instant	¾ cup	223
Shredded Wheat	1 biscuit	3
Raisin Bran	½ cup	209
Corn Flakes	1 cup	256
Rice Krispies	1 cup	340
Crackers		
Saltine	2 crackers	70
Graham	1 cracker	48

FOOD	SERVING	SODIUM (MG)
Convenience Foods		
Cake from Mix		
Yellow	1/12 cake	242
Chocolate	1/12 cake	402
Condiments		
Italian Dressing	1 tbsp.	116
French Dressing	1 tbsp	214
Mayonnaise	1 tbsp.	78
Catsup	1 tbsp	156
Soy Sauce	1 tbsp.	1,029
Garlic Salt	1 tbsp.	1,850
Meat Tenderizer	1 tsp.	1,750
Olives, green	4	323
Pickle, dill	1 large	928
Pickle, sweet	1 large	128
Salt/Spices		
Garlic Salt	1 tsp.	1,850
Onion Salt	1 tsp.	1,620
Seasoning Salt	1 tsp.	1,620
Table Salt	1 tsp.	2,325
Basil	1 tsp.	-
Bay Leaf	1 med.	-
Oregano	1 tsp.	-
Parsley	1 tsp.	5
Thyme	1 tsp.	-
Pudding		
Regular	½ cup	73
Instant	½ cup	195

FOOD	SERVING	SODIUM (MG)
Soup – Canned		
Vegetable	1 cup	823
Tomato	1 cup	872
Mushroom	1 cup	1,076
Chicken Noodle	1 cup	1,107
Snacks		
Potato Chips	10 chips	200
Pretzels (twist)	1 pretzel	101
Peanuts, roasted	1 oz.	119
Nuts, mixed	1 oz.	189
Cheese Crackers	1 piece	20
Candy Corn	1 oz.	60
Fast Food (sandwiches)		
Burger King BK Broiler	1 serving	764
Burger King Chicken Tenders	1 piece	90.2
Burger King Breakfast Croissant	1 serving	1,080
KFC – Chicken Sandwich	1 serving	1,060

REFERENCES

A review of interventions to reduce health disparities in cardiovascular disease in **African Americans.** Crook ED, Bryan NB, Hanks R, Slagle ML, Morris CG, Ross MC, Torres HM, Williams RC, Voelkel C, Walker S, Arrieta MI. Ethn Dis. 2009 Spring;19(2):204-8. Review.

Education, Genetic Ancestry, and Blood Pressure in African Americans and Whites
Amy L. Non, Clarence C. Gravlee, and Connie J. MulliganAmerican Journal of Public Health 2012 102, 8, 1559-1565

Wright Jr JT, Agodoa LY, Appel L, Cushman WC, Taylor AL, Obegdegbe GG, et al. New recommendations for treating hypertension in black patients: evidence and/or consensus? Hypertension. 2010;56:801–3. CrossRef

Redmond N, Baer HJ, Hicks LS. Health behaviors and racial disparity in blood pressure control in the national health and nutrition examination survey. Hypertension. 2011;57:383–9. CrossRef

Flack JM, Sica DA, Bakris G, Brown AL, Ferdinand KC, Grimm Jr RH, et al. Management of high blood pressure in Blacks: an update of the International Society on Hypertension in Blacks consensus statement. Hypertension. 2010;56:780–800.

Peters RM, Flack JM. Salt sensitivity and hypertension in African Americans: implications for cardiovascular nurses. Prog Cardiovasc Nurs. 2000;15:138–44. CrossRef

National Heart, Lung and Blood Institute. *Fact Book Fiscal Year 1996.* Bethesda, Maryland. U.S. Department of Health and Human Services, National Institutes of Health: 1997.

Munson Army Health Center. *Food and Drug Interactions* ; www.munson. amedd.army.mil. retrieved June 2004.

Addressing the Health Care Issue of African-Americans. *Hypertension.* www.blackhealthcare.com retrieved July 2004

Roe, D. A., *Handbook on Drug and Nutrient Interactions – A problem Oriented reference Guide.* 4th Edition. The American Dietetic Association. 1989

National Heart, Lung and Blood Institute. *Your Guide to Lowering Blood Pressure – Manage Your Blood Pressure Drugs.* National Heart, Lung and Blood Institute Health Information Center. www.nhlbi.nuh.gov retrieved August 2004

Fighting Heart Disease and Stroke. *Shaking your salt habit.* American Heart Association. 2001

High Blood Pressure. www.reutershealth.com retrieved August 2004

Larson Duff, R. *Complete food and Nutrition Guide.* The American Dietetic Association. 1996

Cardiology Channel. *Hypertension.* Health Communities. www.cardiologychannel.com Retrieved, July 2004.

Jackson Gastroenterology. High Blood Pressure Diet, www.gicare.com/pated.htm. Retrieved, September 2004.

Kennedy, Ron MD. *Fiber in Nutrition.* The Doctor's Medical Library. www.medical-Library.net Retrieved, September 2004

Alternative-Medicine-and-Health. *Hypertension.* www.alternative-medicine-and-health.com Retrieved, August 2004.

Manual of Clinical Dietetics. *Hypertension.* American Dietetic Association. 6th Edition, 2000

Anderson, J. *Potassium and Health.* Colorado State University Cooperative Extension – Nutrition Resources. August 2004

Tsang, G., *High Blood Pressure Diet – the Dash Diet.* Healthcastle Nutrition Services www.healthcastle.com Retrieved, September 2004.

SECTION TWO

HEART HEALTHY RECIPES FOR THE AFRICAN AMERICAN PALATE

RECIPES

The recipes in this section are to be used as handouts for the patients.

BREAKFAST
DISHES

RICH BREAKFAST BISCUITS

2 cups	All Purpose Flour
2 tsps.	Baking Powder (low sodium)
2 tbsps.	Sugar
½ cup	Corn Oil
¾ cup	Skim Milk

1) Stir flour, baking powder and sugar in a medium bowl.
2) Pour oil and skim milk into flour mixture, stir with fork until four is damp.
3) Knead gently on a floured board for about 30 seconds. Pat out to ½ inch thick.
4) Using a biscuit cutter, cut dough into rounds. Place on ungreased baking sheet.
5) Bake at 450 degrees F for 12 to 15 minutes.

Makes 16 servings
*Heart and Soul

Nutrition Information: per serving

K Calories:	90
Cholesterol:	0 milligrams
Total Fat:	3 grams
Sodium:	6 milligrams

INSTANT BREAKFAST PEACH SHAKE

1	canned peach half
3	tablespoons of dry milk powder
¼	cup ice water
½	package vanilla instant breakfast (2 tablespoons)
¼	cup vanilla ice cream.

Place all ingredients in blender and blend well

Makes: 1 serving
Source: Pass the Calories, Please!

<u>Nutritional Information: per serving</u>

300	Kcalories
11g	protein
10g	fat
Trace of fiber	

BANANA FRENCH TOAST

1	whole egg, slightly beaten
2	egg whites
1	tablespoon honey
¼	teaspoon cinnamon
¼	cup skim milk
1	mashed, overripe banana
	Vegetable cooking spray
10	slices whole wheat bread

Heat griddle or skillet to medium heat. In a shallow bowl or pie pan, mix egg, egg whites, honey, cinnamon, milk and banana.

Spray vegetable cooking spray onto the griddle. Dip bread in the egg mixture, turning to coat both sides. Cook on griddle, about 4 minutes on each side or until golden brown.

Makes 5 serving.
Source: Heart Smart Cookbook

Nutrition Information: per serving

187	Kcalories,
4g	Fat,
359 mg.	Sodium,
55 mg.	Cholesterol

HONEY RAISIN BRAN MUFFINS

1 ¾	cups all-purpose flour
1	tablespoon baking powder
1 ½	cups fat-free milk
½	cup honey
2	egg whites
3	tablespoons vegetable oil
3	cups bran flakes
½	cup raisins

Preheat the oven to 400° F. Spray a 12-cup muffin pan with non-stick cooking spray or line with paper muffin cups. In a large bowl, combine the flour, baking powder, and salt. In another bowl, combine the remaining milk, honey, egg whites, and oil until thoroughly mixed. Add dry ingredients, bran flakes, and raisins until combined. Portion the mix evenly into muffin pan cups and place in the oven.

Bake 25 minutes, or until golden brown and a toothpick in the center comes out clean. Remove from the pan and cool slightly on a wire rack. Serve warm or cold.

Makes 12 muffins (1 serving each)
Source: Kellogg Kitchens Recipes

Nutritional Information: per serving

180	Kcalories
3.5g	Fat
0 mg	Cholesterol
150 mg	Sodium

FRUITY PANCAKES

1 cup	Fruit, chopped (apples, strawberries or blueberries)
½ tbsp.	Vegetable Oil
1	Egg White
1/3 cup	Rolled Oats
2/3 cup	All Purpose Flour
½ tbsp.	Baking Powder (low sodium)

1) Combine oil, milk, egg white and fruit in a medium bowl.
2) In a separate bowl, mix together the flour, oats, sugar and baking powder.
3) Combine both the liquid and the dry ingredients together and stir lightly. Do not over stir.
4) Coat griddle with the non-stick vegetable spray.
5) Cook at 300 deg. F (medium) heat until pancakes bubble. Flip over and cook for approximately one minute. Serve hot.

Makes 4 – 6 (3" x 3") pieces

Nutrition Information: per serving:

K Calories:	134
Cholesterol:	0 milligrams
Total Fat:	2 grams
Sodium:	13 milligrams

VEGETABLE DISHES

(INCLUDING SOUPS)

EASY GREEN BEANS AND TOMATOES IN HERBAL SAUCE

1 1-lb pk.	Frozen Green Beans
1 cup	Fresh Tomatoes, diced

Sauce

1 tsp.	Olive Oil
1 tsp.	Oregano
1 tbsp.	Lemon Juice
1 tsp.	Lemon Pepper

1) Steam green beans in a pot with a small amount of water. Steam until crisp-tender.
2) Drain well. Add chopped tomatoes to the green beans.
3) Combine all the ingredients for the sauce together in a small bowl.
4) Pour sauce over vegetables and toss until coated.

Makes 8 – ¼ cup servings

Nutrition Information: per serving

K Calories:	21
Cholesterol:	0 milligrams
Total Fat:	0.5
Sodium:	7 milligrams

BELL PEPPERS – CREOLE STYLE

4 whole	Green "bell" Peppers, cut in half
2 tsps.	Garlic, minced
¼ cup	Celery, chopped
½ cup	Onion, chopped
¼ cup	Bell Peppers, chopped
¼ cup	Water or defatted stock
¾ lb	Ground Turkey
½ cup	unseasoned Bread Crumbs

1. Put the bell peppers in a medium pot and parboil or steam in water until soft but firm. Drain well and set aside.
2. Sautee onion, celery, peppers (chopped) and garlic in ¼ cup water. Add ground turkey to vegetables and cook until the meat is brown.
3. Drain off any fat. Stir in bread crumbs.
4. Stuff mixture into pepper halves.
5. Bake in 350 dg. F oven for 20 to 30 minutes. Add a small amount of water to bottom of pan to prevent sticking.

Makes 8 servings.

Nutrition Information: per serving

K Calories:	83
Cholesterol:	12 milligrams
Total Fat:	1 gram
Sodium:	60 milligrams

HEARTY PUMPKIN SOUP

2 tbsps.	Water
1 medium	Onion, chopped
1-16 oz. Can	Pumpkin (unsweetened)
2 cups	Chicken Broth (low-sodium)
½ tsps.	Sugar
1/8 tsps.	Cloves, ground
1 cup	Skim Milk

1. In a 2-quaart saucepan with 2 tbsps. water, sauté onions until softened, about 10 minutes.
2. Add pumpkin, broth, sugar and cloves to saucepan, mix well.
3. Bring soup to the boil then reduce the heat and simmer for 15 minutes.
4. Remove from the heat and cool slightly.
5. Puree soup in small amounts in a food blender until smooth.
6. Return the coup to the saucepan and slowly pour in and stir the milk.
7. Cook for 8 – 10 minutes on medium high. DO NOT BOIL. Serve hot.

Makes 5, 1 cup servings.
Source: The ADA Family Cookbook.

Nutrition Information: per serving

K Calories:	104
Cholesterol:	1 milligram
Total Fat:	2 grams
Sodium:	32 milligrams

HEART HEALTHY CHILI

1 lb.	Turkey, ground
½ cup	Onions, chopped
½ cup	Sweet Green Peppers, chopped
2, 8 oz cans	Tomato Sauce (low sodium)
2 cups	Red Kidney Beans, cooked
1 cup	Water
2 tsps.	Chili Powder
1 tbsps.	Herbal Shaker #2 (see herbal shaker section)

1. In a large sauce pan, place ¼ cup of water. When the water starts to boil, place the onions and green pepper and sauté.
2. Add the ground meat to the seasonings in the sauce pan, and allow to cook for approximately 10 minutes, stirring occasionally.
3. Drain off excess liquid.
4. Add remaining ingredients.
5. Cover and simmer for 1 hour, adding extra water if needed.
6. Flavor with herbal shaker #2, or the all-purpose shaker

Makes 6, 8 oz. servings.

Nutrition Information: per serving:

Kcalories:	200
Cholesterol:	5 milligrams
Total Fat:	2 grams
Sodium:	28 milligrams

WALDORF SALAD

6 cups	chopped apples (red and green)
2 stalks	of celery
1 cup	of red or green seedless grapes
½ cup	chopped walnuts toasted
½ cup	raisins
1 cup	non-fat plain yogurt
¼ cup	light mayonnaise
¼ cup	fresh orange juice

In a mixing bowl combine apples, celery, grapes, walnuts, and raisins. In another bowl, mix yogurt, mayonnaise, and orange juice. Toss the dressing with the salad ingredients and chill.

Makes 8-10 servings
Source: Eating Well Through Cancer

Nutritional Information

Kcalories	153
Cholesterol	3 milligrams
Total Fat	6 grams
Sodium	76 milligrams

CREOLE OKRA

1 tsp	olive oil
½	small onion, diced
1	garlic clove, minced
½	small green pepper, diced
1	ripe tomato, seeded and coarsely chopped
½ lb.	fresh okra, sliced into ½ inch pieces
1 tsp	dried oregano
½ tsp	dried thyme

Salt and freshly ground black pepper to taste
Pinch of cayenne pepper, if desired.

In a medium skillet, heat oil over medium-high heat. Add onion and garlic and sauté 3 minutes, stirring frequently. Add green pepper and sauté 3-4 minutes. Add tomatoes and okra. Cover and cook over low heat 10-15 minutes, until okra is soft. Add oregano, thyme, salt and black pepper to taste, and cayenne pepper, if using. Cook uncovered about 1 minute.

Makes 4 servings.
Source: American Institute for Cancer Research Website

Nutritional Information: per serving

Kcalories:	39 calories
Cholesterol:	0 milligrams
Fat:	1 gram
Sodium:	7 milligrams

MEAT DISHES

HOT GARLIC SHRIMP

1 pound large shrimp
1 tbsp. olive oil
4 cloves garlic, smashed, peeled or minced
1/2 to 1 tsp. red pepper flakes
dash cumin
3 tbsp. lemon juice
parsley, chopped, for garnish

Peel and devein shrimp and rinse in cold water. Mix olive oil and garlic in glass measuring cup and microwave on high for 1 minute. In a 2-quart round casserole, mix shrimp with oil and garlic, and sprinkle with red pepper, a few dashes of cumin, and lemon juice. Stir to mix and arrange shrimp in circular fashion, thick ends to the outside of bowl. Cover with vented plastic wrap and microwave on high for 3 to 4 minutes, turning shrimp once. Remove when shrimp are pink. Let stand another minute to complete cooking. Dust with parsley.

Makes 4 Serving
Source: The Diabetes Double-Quick Cookbook

Nutrition Information: per serving:

156	Kcalories
5 g	Total Fat
174 mg	Cholesterol
171 mg	Sodium

BARBECUED CHICKEN

3 lbs.	chicken pieces	1	small onion
1/2 cup	tomato sauce	1/2	cup nonfat plain yogurt
1 tsp.	fresh ginger, chopped	2	garlic cloves
2 tsp.	coriander	1/2 tsp.	cayenne pepper (optional)
2 whole	cloves	1 tsp.	cumin seeds
4	ardamom pods	1 tsp.	salt

Remove the skin and all visible fat from the chicken pieces. (I often have the butcher skin the chicken.) Cut 2-3 slits, 1 inch long and 1/2 inch deep, in each piece of chicken.

Place in a casserole dish and set aside. Cut onion into 4-5 pieces.

In a blender jar put onion, tomato sauce, yogurt, ginger, garlic cloves, coriander, cayenne pepper, cloves, cumin seeds and salt. Blend to a smooth paste.

Pour the paste on the chicken and turn pieces to thoroughly coat with spices. Cover with a lid or plastic wrap and marinate in the refrigerator 4-24 hours.

Preheat oven to 400°F. Remove chicken pieces from the marinade, saving marinade. Arrange pieces in a broiler pan.

Bake uncovered in the middle of the oven for 30 minutes. Turn pieces over and brush with remaining marinade. Bake for 10-15 minutes until chicken is tender.

Turn oven to broil. Turn pieces over once again and broil for 5 minutes.

Transfer to a serving platter.

Serve with lemon wedges or squeeze lemon juice over the chicken before eating, if desired.

Source: Diabetic Recipes

Nutrition Information: per serving

Kcalories: 293
Total Fat :   7.2g
Cholesterol: 159 milligrams
Sodium: 551mg

ORLEANS RED BEANS (STEW)

½ lb.	Dark Red Kidney Beans
1 qt.	Water
8 ozs.	Precooked Turkey Sausage (no added salt)
8 ozs.	Precooked Beef Pieces
1 large	Onion, chopped
1 medium	Sweet Bell Pepper, chopped
4 stalks	Celery, chopped
2	Bay Leaves
2 tbsps.	Herbal Shaker #1 (see herbal shaker section)

Black Pepper to taste

Best if Red Beans are soaked overnight.

1. Place beans in a pot with hot water, and bring to a boil, allowing to simmer for 1 hour.
2. Add chopped seasonings (onion, bell pepper and celery) herbal seasoning, black pepper and bay leaves to the pot.
3. If meat is being used, add bite-size pieces to the beans in the pot.
4. Simmer the entire contents in the pot for an additional hour.
5. Serve over fluffy white rice.

Makes 5 – 8 servings.

Nutrition Information: per serving

K Calories:	286
Cholesterol:	40 milligrams
Total Fat:	5 grams
Sodium:	61 milligrams

OVEN BARBEQUE PORK CHOPS

4 - 4 oz. Pork Chops, lean and trimmed
½ cup Catsup, (low-sodium)
¼ cup Water
1 tbsp. Brown Sugar
4 tbsps. Lemon Juice
2 tsps. Shaker #6

(All-purpose herbal seasoning)
Vegetable Oil Spray

1. Evenly sprinkle the pork chops with Shaker #6 and set aside for approximately 15 minutes.
2. Preheat oven to 350 deg. F. Spray the bottom of a shallow baking pan. Place the pork chops in the pan and into the oven.
3. Brown chops for 20 minutes on each side, then drain off fat.
4. Combine all remaining ingredients in a bowl, stir and then pour the mixture over the meat.
5. Cover the baking pan with foil and simmer for 30 minutes.
6. Remove the cover and continue to simmer for 10 minutes more.
7. Add more water if sauce needs to be thinned.

Makes 4, 4 oz. servings

Nutrition Information: per serving

K Calories: 221
Cholesterol: 65 milligrams
Total Fat: 5 grams
Sodium: 40 milligrams

SWEET AND SOUR CHICKEN SALAD

1-1/4 lbs. boneless skinless chicken breast, cooked and cut into 2 inch cubes

1-1/2 cups celery, diagonally sliced

1 cup snow peas, trimmed

1/2 cup red bell pepper, seeded and diced

1 cup apples, peeled and diced

1/4 cup vinegar

1/4 cup vegetable oil

2 Tbs. sugar

1 tsp. paprika

1 tsp. celery seed

salt and pepper, to taste

Combine all salad ingredients. Whisk together the dressing ingredients. Pour the dressing over the salad and serve.

Source: Diabetic Recipes

Nutrition Information: per serving

Kcalories: 249
Total Fat: 12.0 grams
Cholesterol: 60 milligrams
Sodium: 81 milligrams

SOLE ALMONDINE

1-2	tbsp. butter
2-4	tbsp. slivered blanched almonds
1	tbsp. chopped parsley
2	tbsp. dry white wine
1/4	cup chicken broth
2	sole fillets (or flounder) about 6 ounces each

Heat 1 tablespoon of butter on high in an 8-inch square browning pan a few seconds.

Add almonds and parsley and stir to blend. Cook on high for one minute. Remove dish from oven, add wine and chicken broth, and place fish in center of dish. Cover with plastic wrap and microwave on high for 2 1/2 minutes.

Uncover and place on serving dish, whisking remaining butter into almond sauce. Serve with asparagus and light grain.

Makes 2 Servings
Source: The Diabetes Double-Quick Cookbook

Nutrition Information: per serving:

Kcalories:	179
Total Fat:	11 g
Sodium:	221mg
Cholesterol:	51.5 mg

Baked Salmon with Fruit Salsa

1 lb.	skinless salmon fillets, 1 inch thick, (lightly sprayed with non-stick cooking spray)
3 Tbsp.	Herbal Shaker # 3
½ cup	diced green peppers
½ cup	diced red peppers
1 cup cn.	crushed pineapple in juice, drained with juice reserved
1 tsp.	finely grated fresh ginger

- (Canned Mango or Peaches can be substituted for Pineapple)

1. Line a small sheet pan with non-stick aluminum foil. Arrange salmon on baking sheet. Sprinkle fillets evenly with 2 Tbsp. of Herbal Shaker seasoning #3 blend. Place in pre-heated oven 450°F for about 10 minutes, or until fish flakes easily.
2. Meanwhile, sauté peppers in ¼ cup reserved pineapple juice until crisp-tender. Add remaining Herbal Shaker Seasoning #3 blend, pineapple and ginger. Remove from heat.
3. Arrange salmon on serving plates topped with pineapple salsa.

Makes 4, 4oz fillets with ½ cup salsa
Source: Mouth-watering recipes with a Healthy Twist

Nutritional Information Per Serving:

Kcal	190
Cholesterol	54 mg
Fat:	7 g
Sodium:	45 mg

BEVERAGES

BERRY SMOOTHEE

1, 6 oz can   Frozen Berry Punch Juice Concentrate

1 cup   Skim Milk

1 cup   Water

½ cup   Sugar

1 tsp.   Vanilla

Ice Cubes (12)

1. Place all ingredients into a blender
2. Cover and blend until smooth.
3. Serve immediately.

Makes 6, ¾ cup servings

Nutrition Information: per serving

K Calories: 99

Cholesterol: 0.5 milligrams

Total Fat: 0 grams

Sodium: 21 milligrams

CRANBERRY TEA DELIGHT

2   cups Cranberry Juice Cocktail

4   Tea Bags

2   tbsps. Sugar

2   Cinnamon Sticks, short

12   Cloves, whole

1. Place water in a sauce pan, cover and bring to a boil.
2. Put cloves, cinnamon sticks and sugar in the boiling water. Stir to dissolve sugar.
3. Remove pan from heat. Add tea bags to the solution cover.
4. Brew for 3 minutes then remove cinnamon sticks. Brew for an additional 3 minutes. Remove tea bags.
5. Add cranberry juice cocktail to the tea and return to the heat.
6. Allow the tea to reach to a boil. Remove from the heat. Serve hot.

Makes 6, 1 cup servings

Nutrition Information: per serving

K Calories: 6

Cholesterol: 0 milligrams

Total Fat: 0 grams

Sodium: 4 milligrams

SUNSHINE SIPPER

¼ cup	grapefruit juice
¼ cup	pineapple juice
½ cup	orange juice
½ tbsp.	sugar
½ cup	lime sherbet

Place all ingredients in blender and blend well. Pour into tall frosted glasses.

Yield: 1 serving
Source: Pass the Calories, Please!

Nutritional Information: per serving

Kcalories	270
Protein	3 grams
Total Fat	2 grams
	Trace of fiber

STARCH DISHES

HERBAL RICE

2 cups	Water
1/2 cup	Carrots, shredded
1/2 cup	Celery, sliced
1/4 cup	Onions, chopped
1 tsp.	Garlic, Minced
2 tsps.	Shaker #4
2/3 cup	Rice, long grained

1. In medium sauce pan, combine water, carrots celery, onions, garlic and herbal seasoning. Bring to a gentle boil.
2. Reduce heat and allow vegetable to cook for 2 minutes.
3. Add uncooked rice to the sauce pan.
4. Cover and simmer for 20 minutes or until rice is tender.
5. Remove from heat, let stand for approximately 5 minutes then fluff with a fork.
6. Serve hot.

Makes 2, 6 oz servings

Nutrition Information: per serving

K Calories:	145
Cholesterol:	0 milligrams
Total Fat:	2 grams
Sodium:	23 milligrams

Cheryl Campbell Atkinson

ORANGE SWEET POTATOES

1 lb.	Fresh, Sweet Potatoes
1 cup	Orange Juice
¼ cup	Granulated Sugar
¼ tsp.	Nutmeg
1/8 tsp.	Ginger

1. Boil sweet potatoes for 20 minutes, or until cooked but not mushy.
2. Remove from pot and slice length-wise. Place in casserole dish.
3. Mix orange juice, sugar, ginger and nutmeg together.
4. Pour over sliced sweet potatoes and bake in a moderately hot oven (300 degrees) for 30 minutes. Serve hot.

Makes 4 servings.

Nutritional Information: per serving

K Calories:	110
Cholesterol:	0 milligrams
Total Fat:	0 grams
Sodium:	8 milligrams

ORLEANS POTATOES

4   medium Potatoes, peeled and cut in 4 pieces
2   tbsp. Lemon Pepper
1   tbsp. Parmesan Cheese
2   tsps. Parsley, dried
Vegetable Spray

1. Boil potatoes in a medium pot.
2. Bring to the boil, reduce heat and cook for approx. 15 minutes until tender but not over cooked.
3. Remove from stove top and drain.
4. Spray shallow baking pan with vegetable spray and place potatoes evenly in pan.
5. Spray potatoes lightly with vegetable spray and sprinkle with lemon pepper and parmesan cheese.
6. Place prepared potatoes in a 375 deg. F oven for 15 minutes or until brown.

Makes 4 servings

Nutritional Information: per serving

K calories: 101
Cholesterol: 1 milligram
Total Fat: 1 gram
Sodium: 33 milligram

DESSERT DISHES

PEACH APPLE COBBLER

2   cups Fresh or Frozen Peaches, chunks (peeled)

¾   cups All Purpose Flour

¼   cup Applesauce (unsweetened)

1 ½   tsps. Baking Powder (low sodium)

2/3   cup Skim Milk

½   cup Sugar

Vegetable Oil Spray

1. Using the vegetable oil spray, grease a 1 ½ quart casserole dish.
2. Combine flour, sugar and baking powder in small mixing bowl.
3. Slowly stir in milk then add applesauce to mixture.
4. Pour batter into casserole.
5. Sprinkle peaches evenly on top of batter.
6. Bake at 350 deg. F for about 50 minutes. Serve hot.

Makes 4, 8 oz. cup servings.

Nutrition Information: per serving

K Calories: 195

Cholesterol: 0 milligrams

Total Fat: 0 grams

Sodium: 12 milligrams

ORANGE PEANUT TEA CAKE

2	cups All Purpose Flour
3	tsps. Baking Powder (unsalted)
2	tbsps. Smooth Peanut Butter (no salt added)
2	Egg Whites
1/3	cup Skimmed Evaporated Milk
1/3	cup Water
½	cup Orange Marmalade
½	cup Brown Sugar

1. In a large bowl, sift flour and baking powder (unsalted) and then combine the sugar.
2. Cut in the peanut butter to this flour mixture.
3. In a small bowl, place the milk and the egg. Beat egg mixture with a fork until thoroughly blended and then add to the flour mixture.
4. Beat for 30 seconds with spoon until well blended.
5. Pat into greased 8" x 11" x 1 ½" baking pan.
6. Bake in preheated hot oven at 400 degrees for 25-30 minutes.
7. Serve warm or cold.

Makes 12 (3" x 3") pieces

Nutrition Information: per serving

K Calories:	160
Cholesterol:	0 milligrams
Total Fat:	2 grams
Sodium:	20 milligrams

QUICK AND EASY BROWNIES

1/3	cup butter or margarine; melted
1	cup sugar
1/3	cup cocoa (unsweetened)
2	egg, lightly beaten
¼	tsp. salt
¾	cup flour
½	tsp. baking powder
1	tsp. vanilla

Preheat oven to 350oF.
Grease an 8 x 8- inch baking pan.

In a large saucepan, melt butter. Remove pan from heat and add sugar, cocoa and beaten eggs.

Stir together with a wooden spoon. Stir in salt, flour, baking powder and vanilla.

Spoon into baking pan.
Bake for 20 to 25 minutes. Do not over bake.
Brownies will appear soft and gooey in the middle.

Makes 12 (I bar per serving)
Source: the Cancer Survival Cookbook

Nutrition Information: per serving

Kcalories:	155
Total Fat:	6 grams
Cholesterol:	45 milligrams
Fiber:	very low

Cheryl Campbell Atkinson PhD, RD., LDN.

Received her B.S. in Food Science and Management from Pratt Institute in Brooklyn New York, her M.P.H. in Nutrition from Tulane University in New Orleans, Louisiana and her Ph.D. in International Nutrition from Cornell University. She is a registered dietitian (RD) and a licensed dietitian/nutritionist (LDN), and a member of both the American Dietetic Association and the American Association of Family and Consumer Sciences. She has worked in private practice as a clinical dietitian in Baltimore, Maryland and New Orleans, Louisiana, and is presently a faculty member at Southern University A&M College, Baton Rouge, Louisiana.